How to Lose Weight Without Being Miserable

Prentice Hall LIFE

If life is what you make it, then making it better starts here.

What we learn today can change our lives tomorrow. It can change our goals or change our minds; open up new opportunities or simply inspire us to make a difference. That's why we have created a new breed of books that do more to help you make more of *your* life.

Whether you want more confidence or less stress, a new skill or a different perspective, we've designed *Prentice Hall Life* books to help you to make a change for the better. Together with our authors we share a commitment to bring you the brightest ideas and best ways to manage your life, work and wealth.

In these pages we hope you'll find the ideas you need for the life *you* want. Go on, help yourself.

It's what you make it

* * *

How to
Lose Weight
Without
Being
Miserable

RICHARD TEMPLAR

Prentice Hall Life
is an imprint of

Harlow, England • London • New York • Boston • San Francisco • Toronto • Sydney • Singapore • Hong Kong
Tokyo • Seoul • Taipei • New Delhi • Cape Town • Madrid • Mexico City • Amsterdam • Munich • Paris • Milan

PEARSON EDUCATION LIMITED

Edinburgh Gate
Harlow CM20 2JE
Tel: +44 (0)1279 623623
Fax: +44 (0)1279 431059
Website: www.pearsoned.co.uk

First published in Great Britain in 2010

ISBN: 978-0-273-72554-1

British Library Cataloguing-in-Publication Data
A catalogue record for this book is available from the British Library

Library of Congress Cataloging-in-Publication Data
A catalogue record for this book is available from the Library of Congress

10 9 8 7 6 5 4 3 2 1
13 12 11 10 09

Text design by Design Deluxe
Typeset in ClassicalGaramondBT-Roman by 30
Printed and bound in Great Britain by Clays Ltd, Bungay, Suffolk

The publisher's policy is to use paper manufactured from sustainable forests.

To Elie, a true friend and an inspiration

Contents

Introduction

So you've decided it's time to lose some weight? Good for you. Are you going on a particular diet, or just minding what you eat? Well, either way, the most important thing to grasp is that the key to successful dieting is in your head, not in your stomach.

This book isn't a diet. It's a collection of principles that you can apply to *any* diet in order to make it more effective. Or you can use it as a stand alone without even going on a specific diet.

You can pick bits out of the book that you think will work for you, or you can gradually incorporate the principles one or two at a time until you're using all of them. They'll all help you to lose weight, and to keep it off, without asking you to suffer miserably while everyone around you is merrily eating all the things you're missing.

No, of course I haven't found some magic solution that will allow you to eat a diet of cream cakes and fry-ups without putting on weight. Of course you'll need to consume fewer calories, but the trick is to find ways of doing it that you're happy with.

I have some experience of this myself. When I was young I could eat what I liked and stay as thin as a rake. Then one day I looked in the mirror to find that my entire body had been removed and replaced with an overweight version when I wasn't looking. I still don't know how it happened.

Over the years I tried this diet and that diet, and at my heaviest I was several stone overweight. Then I started to look at other people around me. I wondered why the slim people stayed slim, and what the successful dieters had done that I hadn't.

And I slowly came to realise that all my diets were focused on what I was eating, but the successfully slim people weren't just eating differently from me – they were *thinking* differently. So I set about discovering the kind of thinking that lay behind losing weight successfully, and lo and behold I learnt tricks and strategies that enabled me to lose weight too. I'm now, according to all the medical guides, a healthy weight for my height, and I have vastly more energy than I used to have.

So this book is a collection of all those smart thinking ploys that I learnt from friends and colleagues that make losing weight easy and fun. Yes, I did say fun. It's certainly fun standing on the scales and finding you weigh a great deal less than you used to.

As far as the practical side of dieting is concerned, there's really no getting away from the fact that the bottom line is about burning off more calories than you're consuming. All that guff about calorie-counting diets not working is rubbish. Of course they work (if you stick to them). How can they not work? The science is unarguable.

Sure, your body may start burning fewer calories if you let it think there's a famine going on, but that's only a minor blip in the figures. It can't help burning calories every time you move or breathe. So you'll find throughout the book that while there are no eating plans or calorie listings – this isn't a diet book, as I said – there are plenty of references to the basic calories in/calories out equation.

So what are you waiting for? You've got the resolve and the determination, now let's make sure you have the strategies you need too.

I'm always fascinated to hear of any other ideas for thinking yourself thin, so if you have any great ideas to pass on, or if you want to comment on this book, you can email me at **Richard.Templar@ RichardTemplar.co.uk**.

Good luck!

Richard Templar

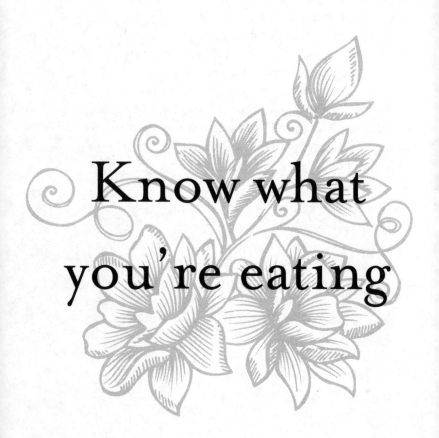

Know what
you're eating

L ook, I hate all that calorie-counting stuff. It really isn't me. And I'm not going to bang on about it for the rest of the book, so don't worry. Nevertheless, I have to concede that those nasty extra pounds build up on account of consuming more calories than we need. So it's worth getting to grips with the basic equation:

3500 calories = 1 lb body fat

Why am I telling you this? Well, partly because if you want to burn off a pound of fat, that's 3500 calories you have to burn up (about seven hours of jogging or aerobics).

And also because for every 3500 unnecessary calories you consume, you'll put on a pound of weight.[1] Let me tell you something. The average weight gain over the Christmas period is 5 lb. Since this weight goes on over about four weeks, that's equivalent to eating about 500 extra calories a day. Or two mince pies.

All those snacks and snippets of food add up, and you need to know this while you're eating them. If you can burn them off again, that's fine. But I presume if you're reading this book that things don't always work out like that.

So as you work your way through the book, just keep this figure in mind – so you can improve your own figure.

[1] Unless you promptly burn it off, of course.

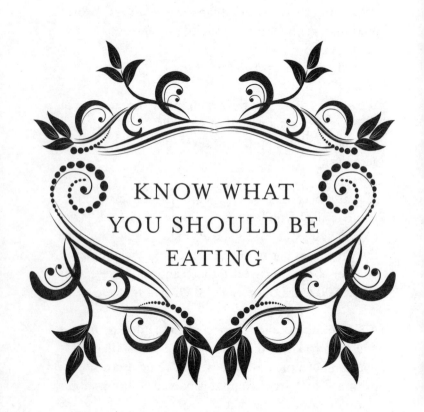

KNOW WHAT
YOU SHOULD BE
EATING

I hope that bit of information in the last tip was helpful. It will be a lot more helpful if you know what you should be aiming to eat. So here is your recommended calorie intake if you have normal levels of activity and no health problems that affect the way you gain and lose weight. Once we've just done this bit, I'll shut up about calories, OK?[1] Obviously everyone's lifestyle, not to mention height and build, is different, so these figures are an approximate guide:

Men	2500 calories
Women	2000 calories

In order to lose weight at the rate of 1lb a week you need to reduce your calorie intake by 500 calories a day (that's what we were looking at in the last tip). So if you're dieting you should aim for roughly:

Men	2000 calories
Women	1500 calories

That assumes that your exercise levels remain the same. Of course you can increase the weight loss if you burn up additional calories.

Obviously you could go on a crash diet, but it's generally inadvisable to eat less than a minimum of 1200 calories a week for women or 1500 for men, unless you're under medical supervision. Best to see a doctor if you want to go on a very low calorie diet, as it becomes difficult (though not impossible) to get all the nutrients you need from your diet.

[1] Well, mostly.

It's a mindset

The problem with diets is that you spend your whole time thinking about food. When can I next eat? Can I get away with one biscuit? How many calories have I got left today? In fact, the trick to losing weight is not to think about food at all, except when you're eating – healthily and in moderation, of course.

Now that's easier said than done. All I can tell you is that it's a state of mind that you need to search for. Once you've found it, get into the groove. The more often you inhabit this state, the easier it will become to get into it. Lots of the suggestions in this book will help you, but in the end you have to find that space in your head which does it for you. It's almost like meditation.

Think of it like this. If you're not a mountaineer, you're not plagued by obsessive thoughts about mountains you're not climbing, are you? So you want to learn to *not* think about eating, along with not swimming or not playing dominoes or not ironing underwater or all the other 'not' things that aren't happening today. Don't think food, don't see food, don't have anything to do with food, except at the 'proper' time. When you finally discover that 'not eating' place in your head, you'll understand exactly what I mean.

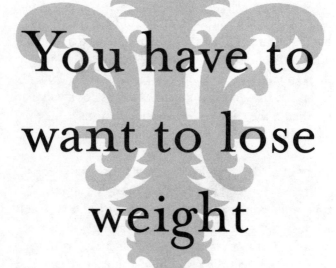

You have to want to lose weight

I tried several times to give up smoking but never quite managed it. The trouble was I didn't really want to give up deep down. I just wished I wanted to – felt I ought to want to. One day, while I was having a smoke, I had an epiphany. I suddenly knew that I truly didn't want to be an addict any longer. And I stubbed out the fag halfway through and never smoked again. I knew this time it was going to work because in the past I'd always told myself, 'I'll just have one last cigarette before I stop,' or, 'I'll give up on 1 January.'

The same goes for getting serious about losing – or controlling – your weight. It's not going to work until you want it right now. Until then, the motivation isn't there in sufficient strength to make it happen. Planning to go on a diet sometime in the future just shows you're not ready yet.

The moral of all this is that you need to find the motivation before you bother with anything else. I can't tell you where it is because it's different for everyone – maybe it's in the sight of yourself naked in the mirror, or in your jeans getting too tight, or in a small child asking why you're so fat, or in the dream of looking good on the beach on your next holiday. It's in all of these for some people, and elsewhere for others. If you haven't yet found it, search for the motivation before you waste your money on lettuce and low calorie snacks.

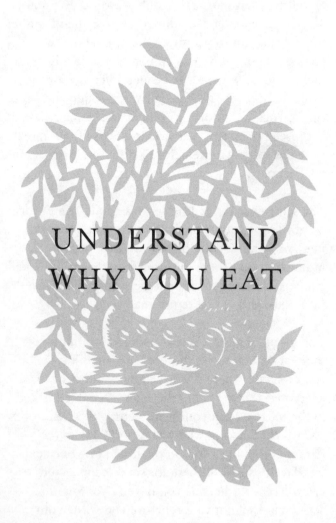

UNDERSTAND
WHY YOU EAT

On the face of it, this is obvious. You're hungry. But if you weigh more than is healthy, that's not the only reason. If you only ate to sate your hunger, you'd never eat more than you need. So what else is causing you to eat?

There are lots of other reasons why people eat. Here are just a few. Maybe you eat when you're:

- bored
- depressed
- lonely
- in a habit of eating at that time
- angry
- feeling bad about yourself
- asserting your independence
- filling an emotional gap.

Most of these are, broadly speaking, negative feelings, and eating may seem to help in the short term, but the long term weight gain will make you feel worse. Overeating is a psychological not a physical problem and in order to tackle it you need to understand the cause. There may be several reasons why you eat when you're not hungry, or different reasons at different times. Until you identify them you won't really get to grips with losing weight without being miserable.

Only eat when you're hungry

It follows on from the last point that you need to make it a rule that you will not eat unless you're hungry. If you're hungry, you'll have stomach pains and you might feel light-headed or queasy or tired. You'll know it's a while since you last ate, and you haven't had much to eat today.

Learn to listen to whether you're actually hungry or not. If you don't have these symptoms, don't eat. I know this is much easier said than done for many of us, but it's an important aim, and at least if you're eating when you're not hungry, you should know that's what you're doing.

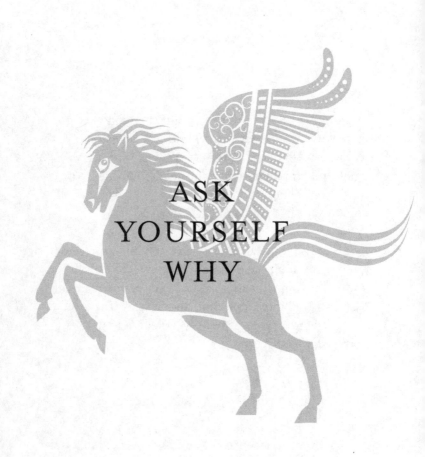

ASK
YOURSELF
WHY

As you reach for that snack, or that second helping, or all those crispy roast potatoes, you should start to recognise when it's not hunger that's driving you. So what is?

Get into the habit of asking yourself why you're eating every time you put food in your mouth. Sometimes the answer will be hunger, but often it will be something else. This is your best opportunity to get to the bottom of why you eat more than you need.

We've already established that there are lots of possible reasons for eating when you're not hungry. So which ones drive you? Are there patterns you can detect? Certain things that spark you off – when you're bored? When you've just come off the phone to your mother-in-law? When your partner puts you down? When you're nervous about a presentation at work? Do you always do your extra unnecessary eating at certain times of the day? Do you always have two biscuits with your morning coffee?

You can see this as a kind of research. Every time you reach for food, ask yourself why. And the answers will build into a picture of when and why you overeat. And that's the ammunition you need to start tackling the problem.

CHANGE YOUR HABITS

Some of the most difficult eating patterns to change are the ones that have become habit. Like always buying a bar of chocolate when you fill up at the petrol station. Or always having a biscuit to dunk in your morning coffee. Yes, I know a biscuit with your coffee is lovely, but there are other ways to enjoy life.

One of the first things you can do is to work out how those calories add up over a year, and translate that into weight gain. For example, one digestive biscuit contains around 70 calories (it varies of course depending on the brand – that's the figure for my personal favourites). If you eat two every day, that comes to 730 biscuits or 51,100 calories a year. That equates to 14 lb of extra weight. That may help motivate you to break the habit.

The easiest way to break habits is to avoid the action that sparks them off. Find a petrol station where you can pay at the pump instead of going into the shop. If you can't resist biscuits with your morning coffee, give up the coffee. If everyone in the office has cakes on a Friday morning, say no and pick that time to be elsewhere – arrange a meeting, do some photocopying, I don't know, just be inventive about it.

Sometimes you'll only need to do this for a while until the habit is broken, and sometimes you might choose to make the change permanent. That's up to you. So long as you break the extra food habit it doesn't matter how you pay for your petrol.

SET GOALS

If you don't know where you're going, you're a lot less likely to arrive there. It's as simple as that. If you're serious about losing weight, set yourself a target.

You might decide to lose a pound a week. Or to weigh half a stone less by the end of next month. Or to feel comfortable in your swimsuit on the beach by the time you go on holiday in August. Or to fit into those jeans you used to wear. Or to be able to run up stairs comfortably. Or to be a particular size in time for your wedding.

The more specific your goal, and the more clearly you can visualise it in your mind's eye, the more effective it will be. You need to have a date for it, otherwise you can't tell whether you're on target or, indeed, whether you'll ever get there.

Work out how much weight you need to lose each week in order to reach your goal. If it's too much, you'll get demoralised when you never make it. If it's too little, you'll get bored waiting to get any slimmer. You should be able to manage a pound a week (that's 500 calories fewer a day), and you may feel – especially with added exercise too – that you can manage a bit more.

Have as clear a visual image as you can of what you want to achieve. Pin up a photo of yourself in those jeans you used to wear, or a picture of how you'd like to look (with your head pasted on the top), or of the clothes you want to buy. Keep looking at it whenever your enthusiasm starts to flag.

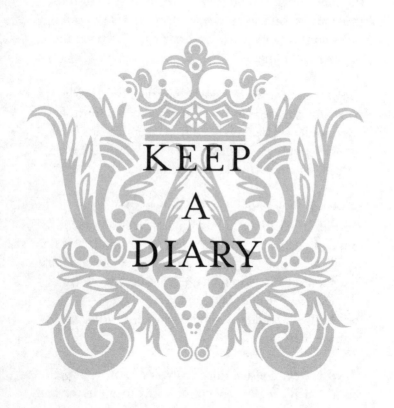

KEEP
A
DIARY

I know it sounds sad, but it works. In fact food scientists report that people who keep a diary of everything they eat can lose up to three times more than people who don't.

There are two reasons why keeping a diary cuts down what you eat. The first is that knowing you're going to have to write it down can be a very good deterrent to eating things you'll regret later. And the other is that if you don't lose weight as fast as you'd like, you can look back at what you've eaten and work out why.

The latest research into this shows that there's an even more effective approach than writing down what you've eaten, and that's to photograph it. Get your phone out and snap a quick photo of your plate before you tuck in. Or of those biscuits or kids' leftovers or sneaky lump of cheese or packet of crisps or whatever else you're picking at or snacking on. Then stick the photos in a scrapbook, or keep them in a file on your computer, arranged day by day.

I can tell you, I think twice about nicking a chocolate from one of my children's stash[1] if I have to photograph it first.

[1] Did I just write that?

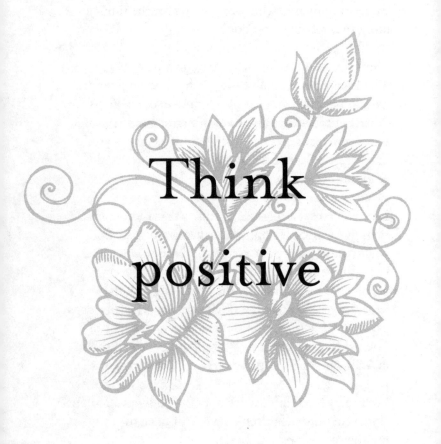

I f there's one thing I've learnt over the years, it's that the psychology of dieting is all important. It should be so easy just to eat fewer calories, but most of us know that somehow it isn't. Those infuriating people who won't be reading this book – so I can safely call them anything I like – somehow do find it that easy. But you and I don't.

What happens? I don't know. We can check out the calories, add them up, make sure they come to whatever we want them to come to... and then we eat a whole packet of biscuits. *Why?*

What I do know is that the trigger is emotional and nothing to do with hunger. And the emotions that can scupper all our good intentions are almost always negative. Anger, depression, boredom, frustration, low self-esteem – they can all drive us to eat.

So one of the biggest things that will help is to get into a positive frame of mind. I know that's easy to say and much harder to do, but acknowledging that you need to do it is important. It means that if you really want to lose weight, you need to sort out your relationship problems, or get counselling, or address all that stuff from your childhood, or at least find an outlet for your negative emotions that doesn't involve putting stuff in your mouth.

Once your outlook is more positive, you still need to eat fewer calories (or burn more of them), but you'll find it so much easier to do.

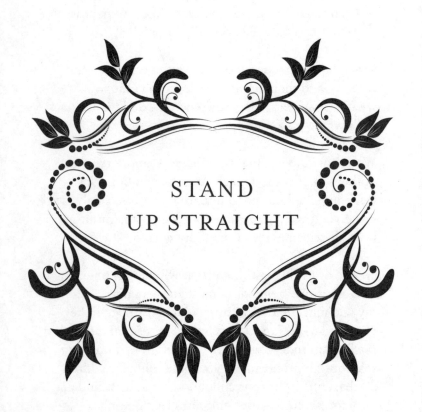

STAND
UP STRAIGHT

Goodness knows why this works so well, but it does. If you sense that your resolve is in danger of slipping – the biscuits are calling, or you've just spotted a particularly succulent sausage left on your child's plate – just stand up straight and put your shoulders back.

This simple, physical change makes it far easier to resist temptation. I'm not saying it's a magic wand and you'll forget the food is there – you do have to do some of the work yourself, you know – but it will stiffen your resolve. At least for long enough to throw the sausage away or leave the room.

At least just try it before you write me off as a madman.

Use affirmations

If you've never used affirmations before, I can tell you it seems pretty pointless. But boy does it work. It's very simple – you just keep telling yourself what you want to hear. Over and over, inside your head and out loud (maybe not out loud when you're in the supermarket queue, unless you're fairly unembarrassable), until it sinks in. And then carry on so that it stays sunk in.

So what are you going to say? Well that's entirely up to you. You might keep telling yourself, 'I can say no to food.' Or, 'I have the willpower to lose weight.' Then again, you may feel the real bar to losing weight is that you eat when you feel unloved. So you could keep telling yourself, 'I am loved and I deserve to be.' Work out what single positive attitude would make most difference to your ability to lose weight, and develop an affirmation to reinforce it. Keep it positive – not 'I'm not going to be fat', but 'I am going to be thin'.

You can use more than one affirmation, but if you try to use dozens you'll just scramble the messages. So start with one or two and, once they take effect, then you can add another.

Eat only
in
public

I don't know about you, but I'm horribly susceptible to the myth that if no one sees you eat something, it doesn't count. Quite why my brain, which I like to think of as being passably intelligent, should fall for such a pathetic con is baffling. Because it wants to believe it, I suppose.

As you see, there is at least a part of my brain that knows it's rubbish, or I wouldn't be writing this. But the gullible part of my brain likes to take over in the face of food, especially when coupled with the opportunity to eat it in private.

The only way around this that I know of is to have a rule that you will only eat in public. I don't mean you have to go down to the town centre with every meal and sit in the middle of the central shopping concourse to eat it. I just mean that you should eat in front of other people, and not when they're out of the room.

Yes, I have spotted that there's a problem here if you live on your own. However, I find that even when I'm alone in the house, making myself sit at the table properly to eat has the same effect. It stops me conning myself into thinking it doesn't count, and in fact, of course, it was only my opinion that mattered all along.

Don't
eat
mindlessly

Here's another eating habit that's really all about attitude. Mindless eating is so unnecessary as to be pointless, but we still do it. You know what I mean by mindless eating – picking at snacks while you're glued to the TV, nibbling on things at a party while you're busy talking, reaching out for another biscuit while you're engrossed in your emails, snacking as you're cooking, eating the leftovers while you clear the table, just because they're there.

This is pointless because not only do you not need the calories, but also you're not actually even enjoying the food. If you want to lose weight, it makes sense to start by cutting out all the food you're not even noticing yourself eat.

The title of this book is *How to Lose Weight **Without Being Miserable***. Well this is the perfect approach then – how can you be miserable about giving up something you weren't really even aware of? Why not make it a rule that you'll only eat food if you're concentrating on enjoying it? That's got to make sense, and it's got to be pretty easy too.

DON'T LISTEN
TO THE
VOICE OF
DOUGHNUTS

There's a little voice inside you – I like to think of it as 'the voice of doughnuts' – which will try to persuade you to eat when you don't need to. It's easy to make the mistake of thinking that this is your voice, that your own body is telling you to eat, but you'd be wrong. This is an alien voice, whose sole purpose is to trick and cajole you into eating food you don't need.

It will come up with all sorts of reasons to have a second helping, or to eat a large piece of cake when a small one – or none at all – would do fine. Just open the fridge door and listen and you'll hear it. It will tell you that 'just one won't hurt', or 'you may not get another chance to eat for a few hours', or 'it'll go off if no one eats it', or 'you haven't had much to eat today'.

Listen out for the voice of doughnuts, and when you hear it start to talk to you, tell it firmly that you're not on speaking terms with it. Cut off diplomatic relations. Recognising the voice, and separating it from your own thoughts, is half the battle won.

DON'T
BELIEVE
THE MYTHS

The voice of doughnuts is very fond of promulgating myths that encourage you to eat when you don't need to. It will tell you that this snack or that second helping 'doesn't count'. You need to learn to recognise these myths for what they are – propagandist twaddle designed to defeat you in your fight against fat.

Just to be sure you know what I'm talking about, here are a few examples of myths you shouldn't be taken in by:

- If it's good for you, it doesn't contain any calories.
- Food eaten off other people's plates contains no calories.
- If it would be rude to decline, the food won't put any weight on you.
- If you eat it standing up, it doesn't count.
- Anything you eat for medicinal purposes, such as chocolate to keep you awake while driving, has no calories.
- If you resist the most fattening thing on the menu, nothing else will put any weight on you at all.
- Anything you eat when you're ill doesn't count.
- If you eat while you're walking, you'll lose weight.
- If you choose something from the menu that is less fattening than what the person you're with is eating, it won't have any calories.

I know these seem as daft as they are when they're written down, but it's surprising how often we allow ourselves to be taken in by them. Along with more plausible, but equally tricksy, arguments such as, 'Just one won't hurt...' or 'I deserve it...'.

SPOT THE TRIGGER

D o you find it hard to have just one chocolate? Or maybe just one slice of bread? Funny, I find I don't struggle at all to have just one apple. Or even just one roast chicken leg. Certain foods tend to trigger a feeding frenzy while others don't.

Not everyone has these danger foods, but most of us do. They're different from one person to the next, but there are some that crop up frequently: bread, pasta, rice, potatoes, grains, cereals – all high carbohydrate foods you'll notice. Cheese is another common one (yep, I can vouch for that) and, no surprises here, chocolate. All those salty things too, like peanuts and crisps.

If you want to lose weight, you'll do well to identify which foods spark you off and eat away all your good intentions. Monitor which things you find hardest to say no to once you've started, and be on the lookout especially for those high carbohydrate, high salt and high sugar foods.

Right then, what are you going to do about it? Well, that's your choice of course, but if you're stuck for ideas I'd suggest you don't keep your danger foods in the house, or only allow yourself to eat them on certain days.[1] Or perhaps be especially firm about not eating them in private. Once you recognise the problem, you're halfway to overcoming it.

[1] No, not any day apart from the third Tuesday in the month. I meant only at weekends, or only when you're eating out.

SPOT THE TRIGGER
(AGAIN)

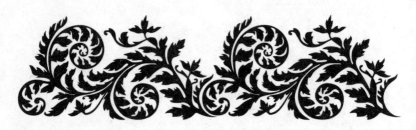

It's not only certain foods that can set off an eating binge. Certain situations and feelings can have the same effect. This can be a matter of habit, such as buying a snack when you pay for your petrol – we've looked at that already – or it might be that when someone upsets you, you reach for the biscuits. Or perhaps you always want food you don't need when you get home from work, or when you're stressed, or when you're bored, or worried.

Once you've identified these danger moments, you can come up with an alternative. Maybe you could start taking a shower when you come in from your dog walk, or phone someone when you're feeling lonely, instead of reaching for food. Perhaps some positive affirmations would help, or just finding something to do to distract yourself. I find that I never stop in the middle of a crossword or sudoku – even for food – so a little book of these by the sofa helps to distract me from eating.

If you try one of these and it doesn't work, don't fret. Just try something different. You'll find an alternative that works sooner or later.

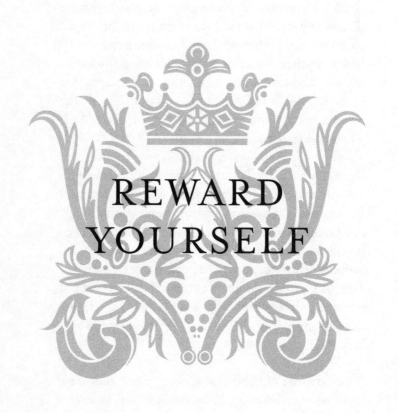

REWARD
YOURSELF

I'll tell you one of my problems when it comes to losing weight – and I've talked to lots of people who tell me they do the same thing: as soon as I lose a couple of pounds I feel so pleased I reward myself. With chocolate.

Thank you, I don't need you to write in and tell me where I'm going wrong. I've worked it out. And actually there are two reasons why my system doesn't work. One is the obvious fact that I'm eating extra calories and undoing the good work. The other is that so long as food and rewards are inextricably linked in your mind, you'll always struggle. It won't only be weight loss for which you'll reward yourself with food. It will be pudding as a reward for eating all your veg, or a slap-up meal as a reward for getting through that presentation at work, or an extra large G&T for surviving your child's birthday party in one piece.

Of course you deserve a reward when you lose weight. Quite right too. So give yourself a trip to the cinema, or a shopping trip, or a candlelit bath, or a massage.[1] Anything really that doesn't involve food.

[1] Obviously I don't mean give *yourself* a massage.

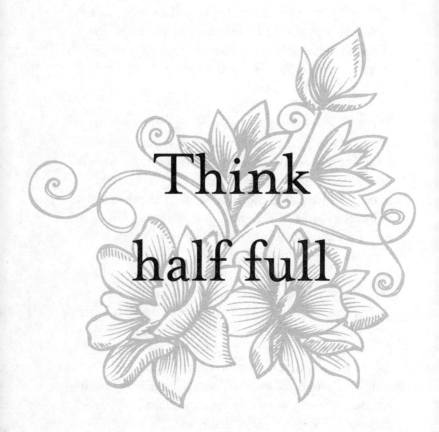

Think
half full

You'll never succeed in losing weight if you're not enjoying it. Once you get underway you should enjoy seeing the scales go down every time you stand on them, but until then you really need to find a way to be positive and upbeat about the whole thing. Researchers have found that people who approach a diet in a more positive frame of mind are more likely to succeed, which is hardly surprising really, but it's nice to know the scientists are keeping up.

One thing you can do is to make sure you focus on what you *can* eat, not what you can't. Don't tell yourself, 'No bread or potatoes for me again tonight.' Instead think, 'Ooh, I've got my favourite soup for supper.' Don't look at what other people have on their plates that you haven't got. In fact, just don't look at what other people have on their plates. Look at the food on your own plate and think, 'Great, I can have loads of broccoli, and that's my favourite.'

In other words, a positive state of mind will add incalculably to the likelihood of getting your weight where you want it. So make sure you don't see the plate as half empty, but be a 'plate half full' person.

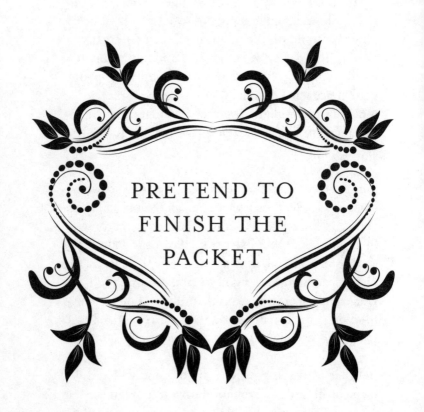

PRETEND TO
FINISH THE
PACKET

OK, this works better for some people than others, and it can take practice. But it's a good mental strategy if you're one of those people who can eat a whole packet of biscuits (or anything else) in one sitting. And I can't deny there's something subversively satisfying about eating a whole packet of biscuits at once.

It's funny, it's so hard not to have another biscuit once the packet is open. It just calls to you until you eat it – which you do of course just to shut it up really. Once the packet is finished though, it's easy to stop.[1] You don't even think about it. The biscuits (or whatever they were) don't call any more.

What you need to do is harness the state of mind that you have after the packet is finished, and get into it after eating only a couple of biscuits. Put the packet away and pretend it's finished. Yes, I know that you know it isn't really finished. But I also know that you know what it feels like once a packet *is* finished. So try feeling like that now.

This might not work the first time you try it. But if you concentrate on your mental state after finishing all the biscuits – until you know it well enough to replicate it any time – you should find that eventually it gets easier to forget the biscuits without having to finish them off first.

[1] Assuming you haven't got another packet in the cupboard.

Meet the family

This is where I make anyone who has ever studied transactional analysis (or TA) cringe with a scarily simplistic summary of what are known as ego-states. But I don't care. We're only concerned with losing weight here, and this should be enough to help you along a little.

According to this system, we adopt one of three states (almost all of us use all three at different times). We behave variously as what is known in TA as parent, adult or child. In fact there's more than one version of each of these. Your 'inner parent', as you might call it can be either a nurturing parent ('You need a nice big bowl of macaroni cheese'), or a critical parent ('You shouldn't have eaten that. It's no wonder you're fat').

Your 'inner child' has three personas. You can be a natural child, who is happy, loving and spontaneous. You can be an adapted child, who has learnt to absorb trauma and accumulate negative feelings ('I might as well be fat, no one cares anyway'). Or you can be a rebellious child ('I'll eat it if I want to!').

The adult in you is sensible, rational and quite possibly the only one who can stick to a diet. In life generally, we need a balance of these three ego-states, but learning to recognise them can help you control your eating. When your partner says, 'You're not supposed to eat that,' and you find yourself saying, 'You're not telling me what I can and can't eat' as you reach for it, that's your rebellious child talking. The adult is the you who can stand up, put your shoulders back and leave the food on the plate.

When you learn to recognise your parent or child voice encouraging you to eat unnecessarily, you can try to switch into your adult state in order to resist.

It would take a whole book to explain this in detail, but if you know that you eat for emotional reasons when you wish you didn't, I'd strongly recommend you find out more about transactional analysis.

Tell your parents where to get off

We get stuck in some dreadful patterns that get harder to shift the older we get. But we can shift them. And we can certainly make sure we don't impose them on our children.

So what did your parents tell you that still affects the way you eat today – and for the worse? How about, 'Finish what's on your plate'? Even if you don't want it, you don't need it and it will prevent you from losing weight.

Here's another: 'You can't have any pudding if you don't eat your first course.' In other words, sweet, sticky, fatty food is wonderful, and savoury food is a trial you have to endure to earn it. And another: 'Come on, eat it up! I hate waste.' Or: 'Think of all the starving children in Africa.'[1] So you finish off leftovers you don't want rather than put them in the compost or the bin.

To be fair to the parents of my generation, obesity wasn't a problem back then, and they'd grown up during the war. But the tenets that worked then are now just a fast track to being overweight.

The fact is that food you don't want or need is wasted whether it's in your belly or in the bin. The only difference is that at least if it's in the bin it's not putting weight on you. I'm not advocating waste, mind you; it's great to budget to avoid leftovers or use them up in the next meal. But even if you have to get rid of them, don't dispose of them via your mouth.

---

[1] I was frequently told this as a child and could never understand it. How would those poor starving children benefit if I ate all my food? Surely it would be better if I left it, and we could send it to them?

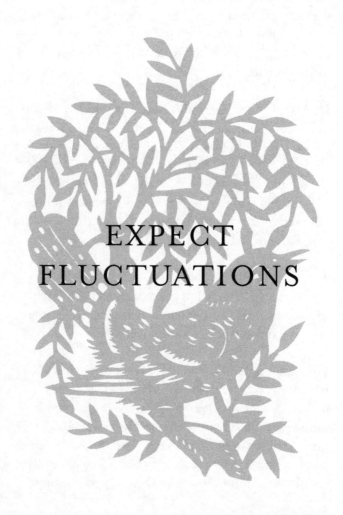

EXPECT
FLUCTUATIONS

Everybody's weight goes up and down. Mine certainly does. You're not aiming to achieve a fixed weight that never alters by an ounce. Sure, you don't want it fluctuating by a couple of stone every few weeks, but a couple of pounds here and there, maybe half a stone over a few months... that's all normal.

So don't be demoralised if you weigh a few pounds more than you did last summer, or if a couple of pounds go back on when you come off your diet. That's nothing to feel upset or worried about.

The object of the exercise is to be able to manage your weight. Not to avoid ever putting on a few pounds, but to have the skills and strategies you need to lose those few pounds when you want to. So long as you're in control of your weight and not the other way round, you're doing fine.

Live on credit, not debt

So it's Saturday night and you're going out for a meal, or treating yourself to a takeaway. Or maybe you're going over to friends for Sunday lunch. Either way, it would be silly to stint on good food, wouldn't it? Where's the fun in that? After all, you can always have a couple of careful days afterwards to make up for it.

Aha! That's where you're going wrong. Because – at least if you're anything like me – those couple of abstemious days almost never happen when it comes to it.

But the solution is really very simple. You're quite right that life's no fun if you can't have the occasional blow-out. So what you need to do is have your couple of days of modest eating *before* you go out. That's right, earn yourself some calorie credits, instead of living in calorie debt. Just think how much more you'll enjoy that meal when you know you've already got credit in the bank.

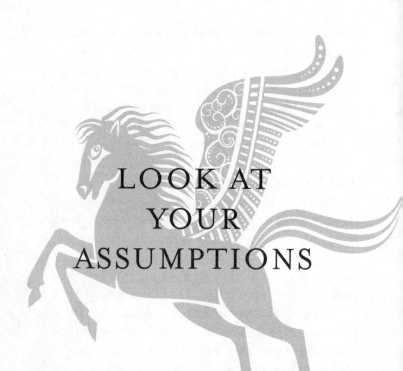

LOOK AT
YOUR
ASSUMPTIONS

When I was growing up, we always had pudding after a meal. It might be light and healthy or it might not. But I just assumed that every meal ended with pudding. Over the years, I've done my best to retrain myself and I now think that pudding is something you have only when you're out or have visitors or it's a special occasion. It's not an everyday thing. This was a long process. For years, after every meal I would think something was missing if I hadn't had pudding. But I got there in the end.

It may be that you have assumptions of the same kind that aren't helping you lose weight. Maybe you don't feel you can start your day without a cooked breakfast. Or perhaps a meal without potatoes doesn't feel right. Or you have to smother loads of things with grated cheese, or eat everything on your plate, or a packed lunch has to contain sandwiches, or tea has to be eaten at 6 pm (so you're hungry again mid-evening).

Try to work out what unhelpful assumptions you have, and work on changing your perception of what constitutes a particular meal. You can always retrain yourself by degrees – I haven't given up puddings for ever, just on the days when I'm eating in without visitors. The key here is really just to identify the problem and take conscious steps to rectify it.

GO ON A PART-TIME DIET

If you have several stone to lose, I'm not sure this one's really for you. But if you just want to lose a few pounds, or maybe maintain your weight but find it less of a struggle, this can work well.

The idea is that you only diet on certain days. Maybe you diet one day a week, or perhaps you diet Monday to Friday and eat what you please (within reason) at the weekend. Or you could diet at home but not when you eat out. This can be adapted to fit round your lifestyle as well as how much weight you want to lose. Aim for an 80:20 approach – diet 80 per cent of the time, and eat normally 20 per cent of the time.

I suspect you've spotted the gaping pitfall here. It's easy to tell yourself on non-diet days that you can eat what you like. If you'd like to try this I'm sure it won't be long before you realise that it doesn't work. That's because people who maintain a healthy weight aren't generally stuffing their faces with doughnuts and half-pound cheeseburgers. You do have to get your head round what constitutes 'eating normally'. In other words, it doesn't mean you can never eat another doughnut (clearly that would be silly), but it does mean common sense and moderation.

If you can do this (and not everyone finds it easy enough to be worthwhile), it's a great way to lose weight gradually without making yourself miserable in the process.

USE PRACTICAL PLOYS

The real battle when it comes to losing weight is in your head. If you don't train yourself to think along the right track you'll never achieve what you want to.

However, there are plenty of practical strategies you can use as well, and you should shamelessly try out every tip, tactic and ploy you can lay your hands on. There are plenty in this book, but don't stop there. Ask around, read articles and come up with your own ideas.

Don't get all sanctimonious about having to do it properly by cultivating the right attitude. Yes, yes, that's quite true, but you need all the other help you can get too, so grab every idea that you reckon has a chance of helping you along the way.

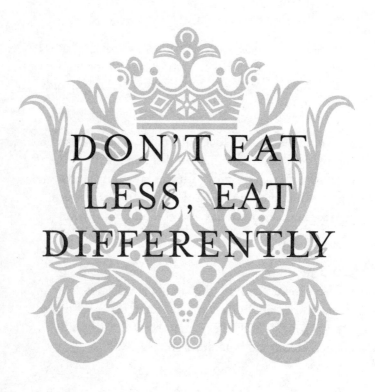

DON'T EAT
LESS, EAT
DIFFERENTLY

The object of the exercise isn't to lose weight by eating less than you do now – although that will work. That would be miserable, which is what we're trying to avoid. No, all you need to do is eat differently.

Sure, if you've a lot of weight to lose you might choose to speed the process up by going on some kind of stringent diet for a while. That's up to you. But you can lose weight just by eating differently, and you'll need to do this to keep the weight off however you get to your target weight.

What's different? Well, food that's grilled instead of fried is different. So is loads of vegetables and a smaller portion of the higher calorie food with it, instead of the other way round. Low fat dressings instead of mayonnaise, lean chicken instead of fatty meat, fruit salad instead of ice cream. You know what the lower calorie options are, or you know where to learn about them.

Keep eating. If you starve yourself you'll lose heart and may give up altogether. And there's no need for it. Just choose foods that fill your plate and keep you eating without adding calories.

IF YOU'RE GOING
TO HAVE A
SECOND HELPING,
DON'T HAVE THE
FIRST ONE

Here's a nice philosophical idea. How can you have the second helping and not the first? I'll tell you. Generally, you know perfectly well when there's a second helping in the offing. Whoever is dishing up will have said something nice and comforting like, 'There's plenty here – everyone can have second helpings.' Or you know your mother always offers second slices of cake at tea time. Or maybe you're dishing it up yourself so you know damn well.

Trouble is, it's so hard to say no to seconds. Well, you don't have to. What you have to do is pass on the *first* round, safe in the knowledge that you'll get another chance. Another bite at the apple pie, so to speak. You have the pleasure of looking forward to your helping, rather than feeling bad about going for seconds, and when everyone else goes for a second round you can say, 'Actually, do you know, I think I will have some after all.'

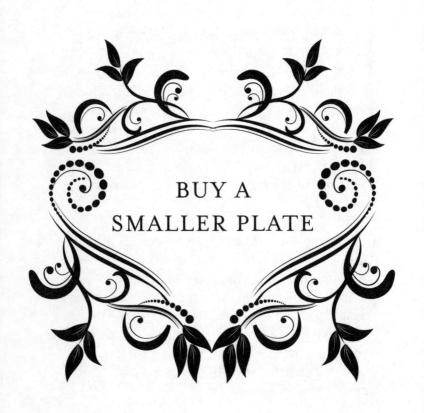

BUY A
SMALLER PLATE

And then use it. If you like the idea of tucking into a plateful of food, piled high and spilling over the sides, you can still do it. You just need to start with a smaller plate. Researchers in the US found that people consumed at least 30 per cent more calories if they had a bigger plate of food put in front of them, even though the smaller plate still had enough food on it to leave them feeling full.

If you have a lot of weight to lose, you might do best with a side plate. If you just want to lose a little – or maybe don't need to lose but would like to fight a little less hard to stay put – buy a plate somewhere between a side plate and a dinner plate.[1]

As a matter of fact, the standard dinner plate size has increased from 10 inches to 12 inches (25 cm to 30 cm) over the last 20 years. It's a good idea to go out to a decent shop and choose yourself a special plate in the right size – possibly an antique shop by the sound of it. If you really like the plate, it will feel special and you'll be much happier to use it. You can even get all possessive about it if you want, and not let anyone else use it. If you find it hard to get excited about shopping for crockery I'm on your side, but I bet there's a plate out there somewhere with your name on it.

[1] No, I don't know what they're called, but I know you can buy them.

Don't finish it off

Make it a rule that you'll leave something on your plate at every meal. It's so easy to feel you have to finish what's on your plate, especially if you were brought up to do so. But if you're not hungry, and you don't need it, why eat it?

Personally I find having a dog helps with this. It makes me feel the food's not wasted as I have someone to give it to (though he's worse than the children at eating vegetables). But, of course, even if it goes in the compost, it's no more wasted than if you ate it when you didn't need to.

I hope you can work out for yourself that leaving one lettuce leaf doesn't really count here. You need to leave something relatively high calorie if you want to feel virtuous.

Of course, over time, and once you've stabilised at the weight you want, it would be less wasteful not to take food you don't need. But that takes practice and this is a useful technique to get you through to that point.

If you
can't resist
temptation,
avoid it

I always used to have the odd packet of biscuits in the house. After all, a couple of digestive biscuits can't do much damage, can they? Probably not, no. Where I went wrong was in cheerfully convincing myself that I was only going to eat a couple of them at a time. Well actually I did only take a couple out of the packet at once. Swiftly followed by another couple, and another, and another.

The way round this is easy. Just don't keep biscuits in the house. It sounds painful, but actually if they aren't there they can't call to you from the cupboard, and you hardly ever think biscuity thoughts. Obviously this goes for crisps, cake, oven chips, whatever your thing is.

And no pretending you have to buy them for the kids. It's much better for them to have the occasional treat than to have chocolate or crisps permanently available. After the initial horror of the new regime, they'll very soon forget there were ever unhealthy snacks in the house.

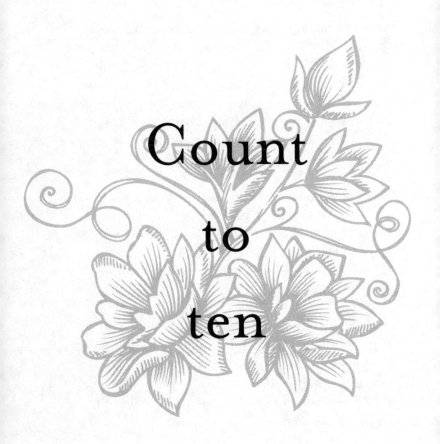

Count

to

ten

M ake it a rule that if you are unavoidably tempted by food, you'll at least count to ten before you pick it up. This might sound futile but actually it's a big help. For one thing, it forces you to stop and think about what you're doing and whether you really want to do it.

You might decide you're still going to eat the food. That's your choice – look, I don't mind, it's your stuff. It's not me that will be putting on the weight. You go ahead, and at least you'll have thought about it and made a conscious choice.

However, you should find that, at least some of the time, just pausing to think is all it takes to stop yourself. Maybe you'll eat something with fewer calories, or maybe nothing at all. The fact that you can stop for a count of ten shows that you could hold off for another ten, and another, and so on until the temptation has passed.

The only thing to watch here is that you don't give yourself a hard time if you still go ahead and eat. Even if this only stops you one time in every ten, you've foregone a tenth of the total calories you'd otherwise have eaten, and you can congratulate yourself on that.

Always shop on a full stomach

L isten, if you're hungry when you go into a supermarket or food shop, you're just asking for trouble. Almost everything you look at can seem tempting – even those revolting pink sweets that appear to be made of expanded polystyrene.

So do yourself a favour and shop straight after a meal. No, it won't work to have an extra snack before you head for the shops. That will just create a whole new problem. Do your shopping straight after breakfast or lunch, or dinner if you must (rather you than me), and you'll find it's much easier to stick to buying the foods you actually need.

Actually, online shopping works well too, although you may not like it for other reasons. If you can stand it, it certainly helps you to stick to the shopping list – making it cheaper for most people even after the delivery charge. A photo of a cereal packet just doesn't tempt as much as those smells they waft at you from the bakery.

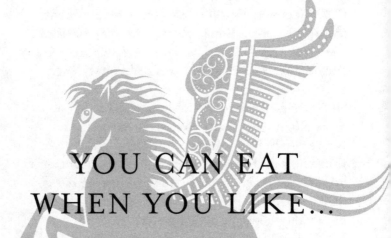

YOU CAN EAT
WHEN YOU LIKE...

There are lots of dieting myths around about when you should eat. Well, take them with a pinch of salt.[1] It's not true that food puts more weight on you at certain times of day. How unscientific would that be? A calorie is a calorie whenever you eat it.

If you really don't want any breakfast, and eating it doesn't work for you when you want to lose weight, then don't eat it. Likewise, if you want to eat an evening meal, please eat one. You don't have to get most of your daily calories down you before lunchtime in order to lose weight, and nor do you have to stop eating at 8 pm.

There are sound psychological advantages for many people in sticking to these rules, but they are not essential and – so long as you don't succumb to the pitfalls – you can disregard them.

[1] Low sodium salt, of course.

...BUT
BE CAREFUL

Now I did warn you that there are pitfalls to avoid if you skip breakfast, or eat in the evenings. So it's only fair to tell you what they are. Then you can make your own decisions about when to eat.

The thing about skipping breakfast is that you risk getting hungry mid-morning and eating a less healthy snack than the breakfast you skipped would have been. If you're at work it will be easy to buy a muffin or a pastry when you could have had a low fat yoghurt with fruit at home. Incidentally, people who eat breakfast also perform faster and more accurately in the mornings according to research, although I agree that's not really relevant to losing weight.

How about the evening stuff? Again, the danger is overeating. We're more prone to snack in the evenings, to eat mindlessly while watching TV and so on, so there's a risk in eating your main meal then. Also, eating in the evening might affect your sleeping patterns, and if you're not getting enough sleep that can tempt you to eat more as well.

Now you know the dangers, you can see why the experts advise you to eat breakfast and not to eat much in the evenings. But if you can resist the temptations then carry on and eat when you like.

ALWAYS PUT FOOD
ON A PLATE

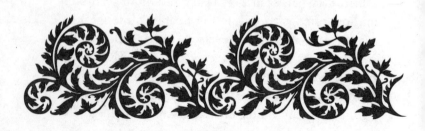

Listen, if you eat straight out of the tin or the fridge or the saucepan or the packet, you'll hardly notice you're doing it. It won't really count, right? Wrong. You may fool your brain, but you can't fool your body. Those calories will get added on whether or not you've personally authorised them.

It's so easy to do – and so simple to stop. Just make it a rule that you won't eat anything unless you've put it on a plate first. It makes you stop and think about what you're doing, and makes you look at it properly and realise what you're eating. And that's often all it takes to pull you up short and stop you picking at things.

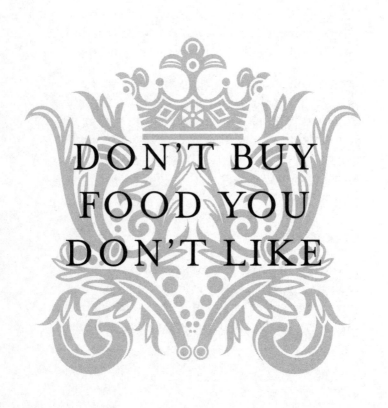

DON'T BUY
FOOD YOU
DON'T LIKE

'**R**ight,' you think. 'I'm going on a diet. I'm going to buy in nothing but salads and low fat foods. No treats, nothing unhealthy.'

I've made this mistake before. You buy in all the things you think you should eat, and forget that actually you don't like salad, or you hate cottage cheese, or you find skinless chicken breasts too dry, or you can't stand cucumber. Then you go to the kitchen to get yourself a nice healthy meal and, surprise, surprise, there's nothing you fancy. So you just finish off yesterday's leftover pudding instead, or go out for a takeaway.

It's all very well being noble, but it won't work. You have to think through what you're going to eat. It's far easier to stick to any kind of diet if you can open the fridge and think, 'Yummm!' So think carefully before you shop about what you actually like eating. Then stick to the low calorie bits of that list, and don't go buying celery just because you think you should.

CHECK WHICH
SNACKS ARE
ACTUALLY
HIGH CALORIE

Here's another mistake I used to make, although I think I've finally learnt now. I used to equate 'healthy' with 'slimming'. So anything that was good for you was OK in my book. I used to snack on nuts, or an apple with a lump of cheese, or raw carrot with houmous.

Of course nuts and cheese and dips aren't actually low calorie at all. They're good for you, and so long as you eat them in moderation you can certainly lose weight if the rest of your diet is suitable. But I wasn't eating them in moderation, because I hadn't grasped just how fattening they could be. Did you know that 100 g of walnuts contains almost 700 calories? Nor did I.

Nuts, cheese, dips, salad dressings, avocados... there are plenty of foods which seem healthy but which can be calorie-packed. So before you start tucking in virtuously, just make sure you know how much of each snack you can get away with eating.

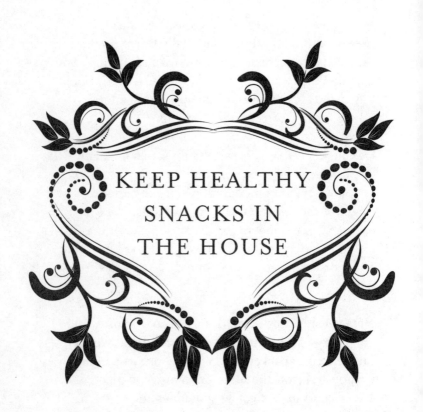

KEEP HEALTHY
SNACKS IN
THE HOUSE

Now you've established which snacks are actually going to help you lose weight and which aren't, the obvious next step is to go and buy them. I know this seems elementary, but actually it's very easy to run out of things, and if you're not an organised shopper it can cause havoc with any plans to lose weight.

It really is important that you make sure there's something in the house you'll want to eat when you need a snack. Otherwise you're bound to weaken and eat whatever you can. Maybe not today, but it's only a matter of time before you have a bad day and, if you can't find any raw carrots, you'll end up eating stuff you know you shouldn't.

Maybe you hate raw carrots. Well sit down (yes now, go on…) and draw up a list of snack foods which aren't high in calories and which you actually like. Then go and buy some in.

Don't buy unhealthy snacks

I may have touched on this elsewhere, but it's worth reiterating. If you continue to keep your old favourite snacks around you, sooner or later your resolve will fail and you'll eat them. After all, why have you bought them unless you're planning to eat them? If anyone else in your family likes them, tough. They'll have to learn to eat celery and cottage cheese instead.[1]

Wouldn't it be great to be the kind of person who can look their favourite snack in the eye and then just turn their back on it? Well, you're not. Not yet. Let's not try to run before we can walk.

[1] Only joking. No one can like celery and cottage cheese. But you take my point.

Make it
a ritual

If you're going to fix yourself a snack, it can help to make a big deal out of it. It makes you feel as if you've eaten properly, compared to grabbing a handful of dried fruit out of a jar.

I have a friend who used to eat onion and tomato salad for lunch when he was losing weight (successfully, I might add). He'd get out the chopping board and the knife, fetch a couple of tomatoes and half an onion,[1] and get a plate ready. Then he'd thinly slice the tomatoes and onion and lay them overlapping on the plate. Then he'd sit down and eat it. You see, although the calorific value was just about nil, and the volume of food wasn't great, he felt as if he'd eaten so could happily go another few hours before eating again.

This is kind of an extension of always putting your food on a plate. It just makes each snack or meal into a more noticeable and significant event, and is more satisfying both physically and psychologically.

---

[1] Before you say anything, you *can* fetch half an onion. It's the half left over from yesterday's salad.

Stop!

One of my kids had a birthday party the other day (all offers of sympathy gratefully accepted). On the table was a bowl of crisps. I so nearly reached out and took one, and then I remembered. I remembered that once you start, it's even harder to stop than if you don't have the first one. So I resisted.

Two days later I was having lunch with a friend. I was having a (delicious) salad while he had a steak sandwich and fries. He kindly invited me to help myself to chips, which of course would have been fatal. I hit on what I thought was an ingenious plan though. I said, 'I won't thanks, in case I can't stop. But if you'd like to leave me the last one or two in the bowl that would be great.' He did, and I thoroughly enjoyed them knowing I couldn't be tempted to eat any more because they'd all gone. (Mind you, he'd eaten all the nicest, crispiest ones himself.)

The moral here is, don't kid yourself you can stop. If you can't stop *before* you've started, you certainly won't be able to afterwards. This is the least hard moment to say no. It goes downhill after this.

On the other hand, if you can wangle the last one or two before they're all gone, you're on to a winner.

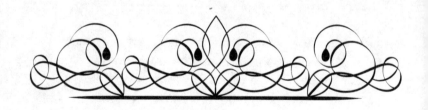

Use

stronger

food

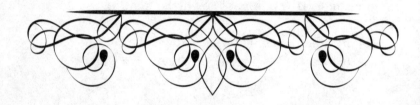

One way to keep your calorie intake down when you're cooking is to substitute strong tasting food for milder flavours. For example, if you flavour your cheese sauce with Parmesan instead of mild cheddar, you'll need fewer calories-worth to produce the same degree of flavour.

Be on the lookout for other useful substitutions. Salted butter tastes stronger than unsalted. Bacon in a recipe will taste stronger than ham, so you can use less. Extra virgin olive oil is tastier than light and mild varieties. Spices add flavour without having to use more fattening ingredients. You don't need me to tell you all the possibilities. Just go through recipes and see if there are any useful substitutions you can make before you start cooking.

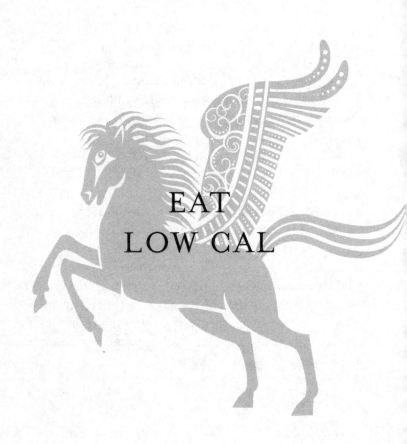

EAT
LOW CAL

It's not only the strength of foods you can substitute, of course. You can also replace high calorie foods with lower calorie alternatives. Low fat margarine can replace butter, filo pastry can replace puff pastry, skimmed milk can replace semi-skimmed or full fat, trimmed back bacon can substitute for streaky, and so on.

It's just a matter of habit. Once you get used to replacing cream with crème fraîche, thick-sliced bread with medium-sliced,[1] white bread with brown, you will find yourself automatically going to a different shelf in the supermarket. Before long your cupboard will contain only low fat mayonnaise, tuna canned in spring water instead of oil, and so on.

In other words, it gets easier as you go on. Just make a bit of effort to learn the right substitutes now, and before long you'll be eating more slimming food without even noticing.

[1] Why can't you buy thin-sliced bread any more? And if you can't, why don't they change the name of medium-sliced to thin-sliced?

BE
LABEL
SMART

They're out to get us, you know. Those food manufacturers – they think they can fool us. But we're not that stupid and we won't fall for their tricks. We know that 'reduced fat' doesn't mean we can eat it without putting on weight. 'Low fat' doesn't mean it doesn't contain any fat. And 'polyunsaturated' or 'monounsaturated' fats contain just as many calories, even if they are better for you in other ways.

Here are some sneaky labelling devices to be on the lookout for:

- 'Reduced fat' just means it has less fat than it used to have, or less fat than the full fat variety. It may still be packed with calories.

- Similarly, 'low fat' doesn't actually mean 'low fat'. It just means low fat *for that food*. Low fat mayonnaise certainly has less fat than normal mayo, but mayo is made with oil and eggs so it's still going to be a high fat food.

- 'Ninety per cent fat free' means that 10 per cent of the food is made up of fat. If you really want a low fat content, look at the values per 100 g, and aim for 3 g of fat or less.

- The same of course goes for sugar, salt and anything else.

The fact is that you have to read the label to find out what's really in the stuff, and don't take any notice of the claims on the packaging.

GRILL, DON'T FRY

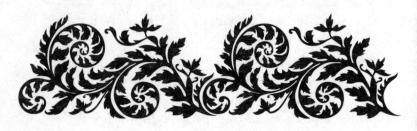

The way you cook your food makes a big difference to how you control your weight. One tablespoon of oil contains around 120 calories. If you cook in a tablespoon of oil five days a week, that's over half a stone's worth of calories in a year. Are you sure it's worth it?

Always grill your food instead of frying it if you can, or bake it in the oven on a rack so the fat can run off. Another simple change that will soon become habit. I used to love fried food, but I actually prefer grilled now as I've grown used to it. I find a lot of fried food too claggy and rich.

Of course, sometimes a recipe does call for you to use a frying pan. And as I don't want you to be miserable, I shan't say never ever fry anything. But what you can do is save up for a good non-stick frying pan so you don't need to add much oil to cook in, if any. Or at least use a spray oil, which uses up far less.

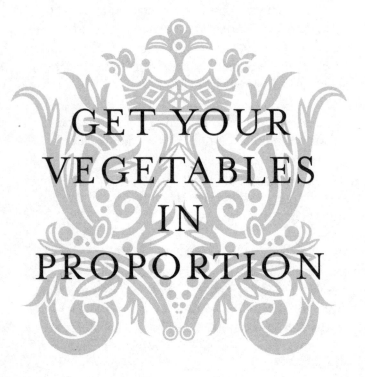

GET YOUR
VEGETABLES
IN
PROPORTION

You're already eating off a smaller plate, I hope (or are about to be). Now you need to think about the balance of foods on your plate. No good filling it up with grilled steak and potatoes and then half-heartedly adding half a dozen peas on the side.

You need to be filling around two-thirds of your plate with vegetables – steamed greens, braised carrots, crunchy salad, you choose. That leaves you just a third of a (smaller) plate to divide between meat or other protein[1] and starchy foods.

Personally I've started cooking much more interesting vegetables now I've discovered I have to eat so many of them. I make tasty salads with sunflower seeds and crunchy apple in them, or I braise cabbage with fennel and cumin seeds, or grate carrot and celeriac together and dress with a little lemon juice. It suddenly seems worthwhile when I've got to stuff that amount of them down me. And the consequence, of course, is that I really enjoy them.

---

[1] Ha! If you're vegetarian you won't catch me out forgetting about you. Fat chance – my editor's a vegetarian.

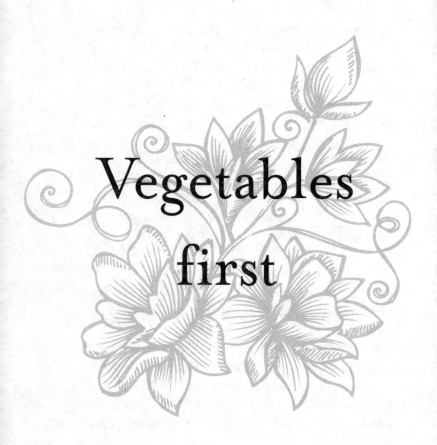

Vegetables first

I know what you're thinking. Once the rest of the food is on the plate, there may not be enough room for the amount of vegetables I've just told you to eat. And you're absolutely right.

Which is why you need to put the vegetables on your plate first. If you don't leave much room for starchy and fatty foods, you can't dish them up to yourself.

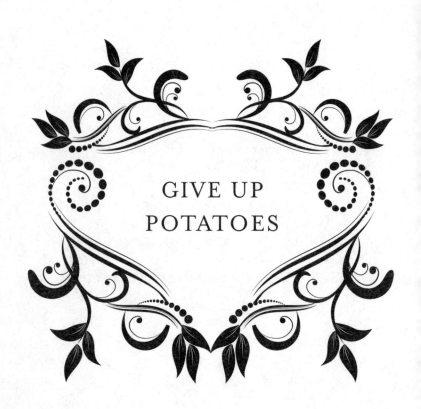

GIVE UP
POTATOES

There's really no point in potatoes. Unless you're on a special diet which requires you to eat loads of carbohydrate, you might as well give them up.

They're not that good for you, you know. The bit just under the skin is really the only part worth having. So although the calorie content isn't that high, you could be getting those calories elsewhere along with other valuable nutrients.

The other problem with potatoes is that there aren't really any ways of preparing them that don't either taste dry and boring or add calories. They can be delicious, without a doubt, but only if you roast them in fat, or drizzle melted butter over them, or top them with grated cheese. Leave out all those things that make them tasty (and fattening) and there's not much left.

So my advice is to give them up. Skip the obligatory portion of carbohydrate on your plate at every meal and just have more of your other vegetables instead.

Never eat anything bigger than your fist

And before you ask, yes, that's your own fist.
No good finding a huge hulking bloke and
borrowing his. Then again, look on the bright
side, you don't have to use a two year old's fist
either.

Look, this whole thing is about moderation, and
your fist is as good a gauge of moderation as any. A
portion of fruit or vegetables is reckoned to be a
helping the size of your fist, so this isn't
unreasonable.

If we're honest, eating a portion of lettuce or
watercress bigger than your fist won't do you much
harm weight-wise. Especially when you allow for all
the air in between the leaves. And if you've left your
salad undressed.[1] This rule really comes into its own
for things like mashed potato, cake, chips, red meat,
steamed sponge pudding,... oh, you know perfectly
well when you need to apply it.

[1] Now, now.

Hands off the kids' leftovers

If you have kids, you'll doubtless be well aware of the temptations of leftovers. Sometimes they look so revolting you wouldn't touch them if you were starving, but sometimes they can seem quite appetising. That untouched fishfinger, those cheese sandwiches, the end of that packet of crisps...

Stop! Have you ever added up how much extra food you can consume in a week this way? And when was the last time you stinted on your own food to compensate? 'I won't have much, thank you. I had half a sausage, three crisps, a soggy digestive biscuit and some grated cheese earlier.'

So what's the answer? How are you going to resist temptation? I'll tell you. You're going to remove it. As soon as the children finish eating, squirt washing-up liquid all over the plate before you have a chance to snaffle anything off it. Or if you prefer, scrape it off into the compost, or the dog's bowl (assuming you won't stoop low enough to eat from these). Better still, train the children to dispose of the leftovers when they leave the table.

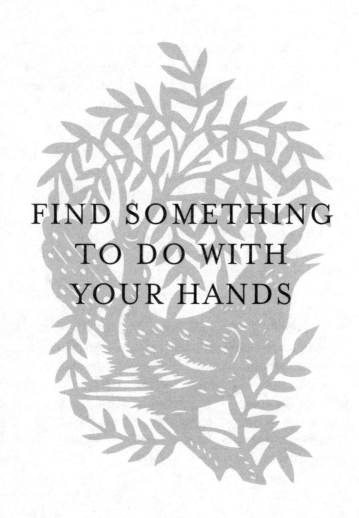

FIND SOMETHING
TO DO WITH
YOUR HANDS

This may not apply to you, in which case feel free to move on. But lots of us – especially those of us who used to smoke – find that eating gives us something to do with our hands. You're sitting around in the evening, your hands aren't occupied, so you fill them with food to keep them busy. If you're an ex-smoker like me, this is an especially good solution as it even involves raising your hands to your mouth intermittently.

When I say it's an especially good solution, what I actually mean is that it's an especially bad solution. It solves the wanting a fag problem, but it creates another bigger[1] problem.

The answer, of course, is to find some other way to occupy your hands. Take up crocheting or sudoku or check your emails or buy a set of worry beads. Anything that keeps your fingers busy so they don't need to drag you off to the kitchen to find them something to do.

[1] Literally.

Distract
yourself

What do you do when you hear food calling you from the fridge or the cupboard? Do you walk zombie-like, with glazed eyes, to the source of the sound? Well, what else can you do?

Anything. You can do anything you like. Just find some way to distract yourself. Make it your automatic reaction when you start thinking about food. Don't sit there trying not to think about it. Do something else. Go for a walk, do some work, challenge the kids to a game of football, phone a friend, clean the bathroom, wash the car, get the laundry done.

In fact anything involving water is generally a good idea. It's almost impossible to eat while you're having a shower.

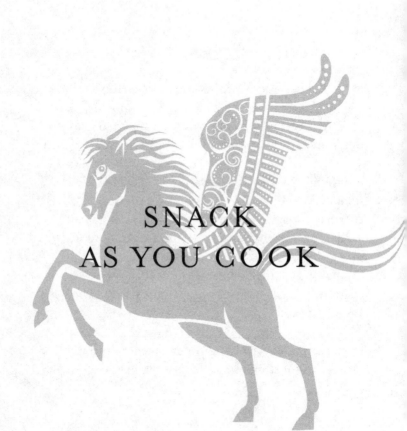

SNACK
AS YOU COOK

I know it's best not to pick at food while you're cooking. You do it almost without thinking, and unless you're making salad or something similar it can scupper your intentions of losing weight.

But let's be realistic here. Sometimes you have to cook and know you won't be able to resist. So rather than kid yourself you'll be restrained and then finding that you give in, the best solution is to have a snack to hand for picking at. Have some apple slices, or a raw carrot, or whatever you need to distract you from the food you're preparing and divert you towards something lower in calories.

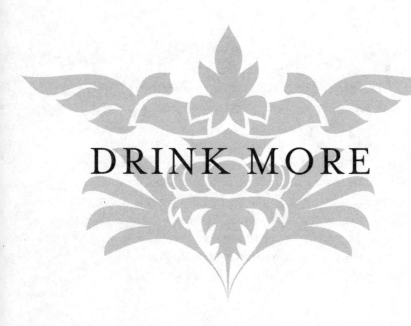

DRINK MORE

I'm talking about water here, before you ask. They say you should drink around two litres a day, which is roughly eight glasses. You might personally find that your own optimum level is a bit lower or higher than this, but certainly if you drink very little you should find that drinking plenty of water really helps you lose weight.

It seems that water helps to boost your metabolic rate, so you burn more calories. It also helps you to flush out retained water, which will generally reduce your weight by a few pounds. And if you are losing weight, your kidneys will need the extra water to help them flush out all the waste products from converting stored fat into energy.

On top of that, drinking water fills you up so you feel less need to eat. If you're feeling peckish shortly before a meal don't have an extra snack, just have a glass of water. And if you're drinking water, you're less likely to drink calorific drinks instead.

DRINK LESS

I hate to tell you this, but then you already know it – drinking alcohol is one of the easiest ways to scupper any diet. A small glass of wine contains about 100 calories. A pint of beer has about 240 calories. So drinking in moderation may be fine – it may even be good for you – but if you're inclined to put away half a bottle of wine a night, just think what that's adding to your weight over a year.

You don't have to become teetotal. Just cutting down will make a difference. You'll probably find it harder to cut down to one glass a night than not to open the bottle at all. So why not have drinking days and non-drinking days? You might take a week off every month, or maybe drink alcohol only at weekends, or only when you're out.

I'm sure you can decide what system works best for you. Just make sure that if you're serious about losing weight, you keep your alcohol intake low.

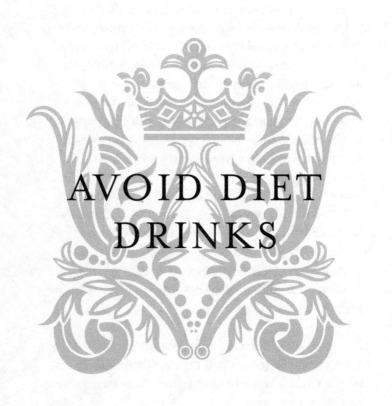

AVOID DIET DRINKS

This seems contradictory. Surely if they're *diet* drinks they'll help you lose weight, won't they? Strangely enough, no. It's quite true that they contain fewer calories than their sugar-filled counterparts, but it's not that simple.

The problem is artificial sweeteners, which these drinks contain in significant quantities. When you consume these sweeteners your body tastes the sweetness and gets ready for a substantial influx of calories. When these don't materialise your body starts asking for them by feeling hungry, so you're encouraged to eat more.

In fact, researchers have discovered that people who drink just one diet drink a day are 30 per cent more likely to become obese than people who don't.

Of course, this doesn't apply only to diet drinks. They're the biggest culprit because they're so sweet, but ideally it's best to avoid artificial sweeteners in other products too.

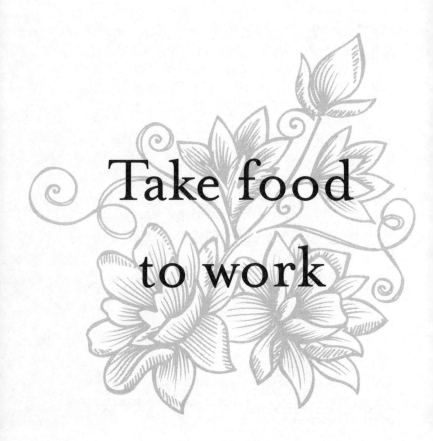

Take food
to work

If you go out to work, you have to eat during the day. And if you're surrounded by fast food outlets, sandwich bars and cafeterias, it's pretty hard to find something really healthy and low calorie to eat. And it can be even harder to make yourself order it when it's surrounded by other temptations.

So take your own food into work. Not only can you control exactly what you eat, but also you won't have to look at all the other tasty things on offer. It's easy enough to rustle up a salad or some raw vegetables with dips, or some cottage cheese with fruit.

And don't start moaning that you don't have time. Look, it's your choice. If you don't want to lose the weight, I don't care. But if you do, you'll find the time. You can buy in ready-prepared salad, or make enough meals for the week and keep them in the fridge or freezer. Or grab a couple of bananas, a tub of low fat yoghurt and a healthy cereal bar. Where there's a will, there's a way.

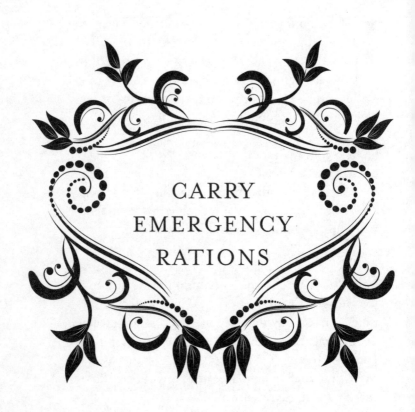

CARRY
EMERGENCY
RATIONS

S uppose you get hungry when you're at work or out and about – what do you do? Ignore it manfully,[1] or relent and buy something you didn't mean to eat? Personally I fall into the second camp far too often.

Suppose you already had a handy snack with you though? You could eat that instead of going and buying a muffin or a bar of chocolate. Now there's a thought.

This is another of those ideas that I'm including because it works brilliantly for some people. However, I'm aware it doesn't work for everyone. If that snack is burning a hole in your pocket, you may end up eating it when you didn't need it and still being hungry later. If this is you, skip to the next tip (the next one can't possibly backfire on you).

However, if you think you could run with this, give it a try. You may find it saves you from all sorts of worse eventualities.

---

[1] Or womanfully.

Weigh
yourself

Maybe you do this already, but if you don't I recommend it. Three-quarters of all successful slimmers weigh themselves at least once a week.

It makes sense. If you don't know how you're doing, how can you modify it when the weight isn't coming off as fast as you'd like? You won't even know. I realise you'll notice when you can't do your trousers up any more – or more optimistically when they won't stay up – but that's a pretty crude measure frankly.

If you want to be able to make adjustments to your diet, and to monitor how you're doing, it's no good burying your head in the sand. It's just crazy to say you want to lose weight and then avoid any means of knowing whether you're succeeding.

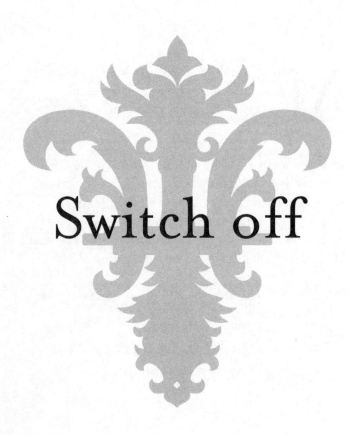

Switch off

Watching too much TV makes it hard to lose weight. Honestly. It's not the TV per se, it's a combination of the fact that heavy TV-watchers[1] take less exercise and the fact that your hands are free to do that mindless eating thing.

Over 60 per cent of people who successfully lose weight watch less than ten hours of TV a week. That's under an hour and a half a day. To be honest, there's really not that much on – surely no one needs to watch more TV than that? Look through the listings at the beginning of the week and pick the things you really want to watch, and turn off the rest of the time, or leave the room. Almost anything else you do will burn more calories, even just cutting your toenails.

[1] In both senses.

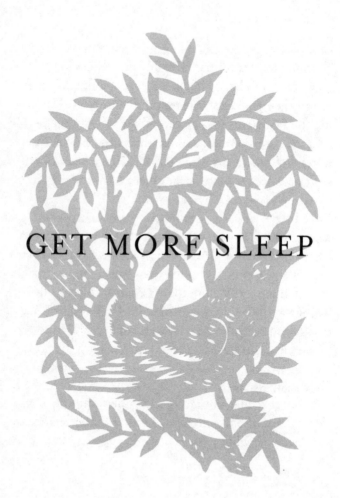

GET MORE SLEEP

If you're not getting enough sleep, it makes it much harder to lose weight. Those busy researcher chaps have been at it again, and have found that if you get less than five hours of sleep a night you're over 30 per cent more likely to gain weight than someone who gets at least seven hours of sleep. If you're getting six hours a night I can't help you, researchers being what they are. They didn't oblige with that particular figure.

The researchers can only speculate about the reasons behind the facts, but their guess seems right – the more tired you are, the more likely you are to eat sugary snacks to keep yourself awake. I don't know about you, but I'd certainly find it hard to lose weight on a regular five hours a night. I'd be eating all day to keep myself awake.

So, if you regularly suffer from sleep problems, see if you can sort that out alongside your slimming efforts, because it will give you a far better chance of losing the weight.

Don't get hungry

Although many of the barriers to losing weight are in your head and not on your plate, it certainly doesn't help if your body is sending messages telling you that you must eat as much as possible right now.

If you feel hungry when you sit down to eat, you're likely to eat as much as you can as fast as you can – within the bounds of modesty and decency, of course. What happens is that by the time your brain has noticed you're full, you're way ahead and have eaten another helping and a pudding, neither of which you really needed.

Far better to make sure you don't get that hungry, and to eat slowly enough that your brain gets the message you're full as soon as you've eaten enough, instead of being several courses behind your stomach.

You'll find some more specific ideas on the next few pages to help you achieve this. If you never feel too hungry – and never think you're hungrier than you are – you won't eat so much.

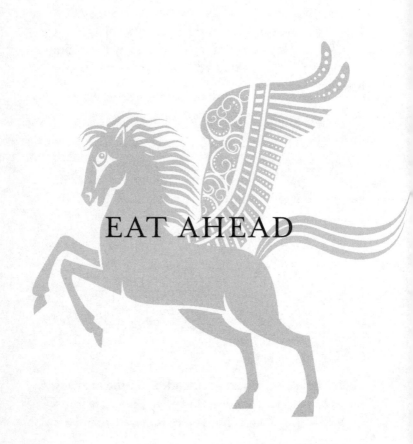

EAT AHEAD

It's much easier to eat in moderation at mealtimes if you're not so ravenous that you cram everything you can down your throat. So it makes sense to take the edge off your hunger before you sit down to eat. That way, you'll find it easier to put less food on your plate, not to mention pinching all the crispiest roast potatoes before anyone else gets a chance.[1]

There's no point trying to reduce the hunger by eating an entire small meal ahead of the main one. That would just be counter-productive. One of the best ways to dampen your hunger is to drink a glass of water about 20 minutes before you eat. It's good for you and dulls your appetite. If that doesn't do it for you, eat an apple.

[1] Or is that just me?

EAT MORE
SLOWLY

The slower you eat, the more opportunity your body has to tell your brain when you're full. You don't want to get ahead of it and wolf down loads of calories you don't need before you've noticed you're not actually hungry any more.

So slow down. I feel a bit hypocritical saying this, since I've never been known for doing anything slowly, but just because I struggle with this doesn't mean you can't get it right.

Try chewing each mouthful 20 times before you swallow it. Put your knife and fork down between mouthfuls. Rest halfway through for a minute or two. The idea is that by the time second helpings are in the offing, or the possibility of pudding, you know that you're not actually hungry. It doesn't solve the whole problem (especially if there are a couple of crispy roast potatoes still left in the dish), but it certainly helps.

Another trick is to cook food that takes longer to eat – picking round the fish bones or munching your way through corn on the cob will slow you down a bit.

PAUSE BETWEEN
COURSES

Unless you're eating at a friend's house, you can generally control the time between courses. If you're eating out, you can always ask your waiter for a break. And in your own house, you can certainly organise your own time.

I'm not just talking about sitting politely for an extra five minutes before you stack the plates and get the next course on the table. That will certainly help your brain catch up with the fact you're no longer hungry, but you can take a longer break than that. Maybe load the first-course plates in the dishwasher or put them in the sink to soak, tidy away all the condiments (that sounds very proper), and so on. Or you could take half an hour and come back later to finish the meal.

If you're prone to snack in the evening, you could split the meal even more. I know one family who routinely have their evening meal at about 6.30, and always have pudding a couple of hours later. They tell me that if they had it straight after the meal, they'd end up eating something else at 8.30 as well.

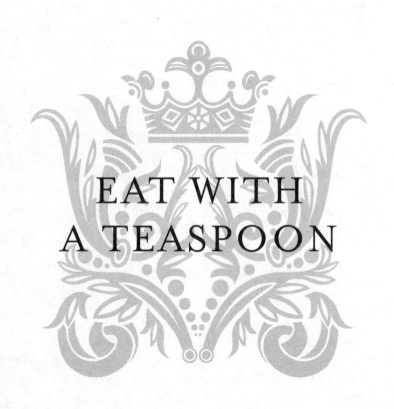

EAT WITH
A TEASPOON

It takes longer.

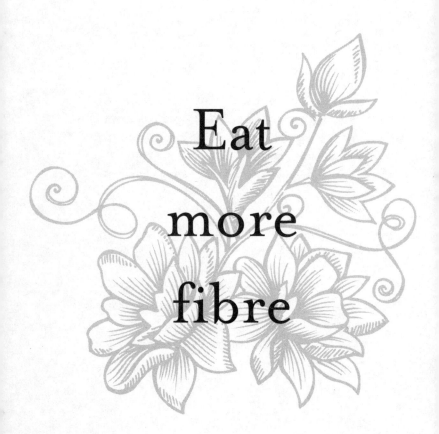

Eat
more
fibre

High fibre foods make you feel full faster, so they help you to stop eating sooner. You'll fill up quicker with wholemeal bread than with white bread, for example (and it's better for you). The same goes for wholewheat pasta and brown rice.

You can take this one stage further. As well as substituting more fibrous foods for what you'd normally eat, you can add (low calorie) fibre to your cooking in order to fill you up faster. So cook with wholemeal flour, and add beans or peas to soups and stews. Chuck a handful of pearl barley in your casserole, or chop up an apple to add to your salad.

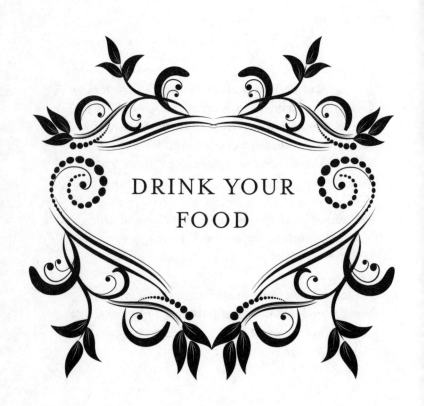

DRINK YOUR
FOOD

Food that has a high water content fills you up quicker and helps you to feel fuller for longer. All you have to do is turn your vegetables into soup, or your fruit into smoothies, and it will help deter you from eating other things.

If you're eating out at a restaurant, order soup as your starter and you'll find it easier to say no to extras with your main course, or to leave food that you don't need on your plate. Or, of course, to pass on pudding.

You can make a great breakfast smoothie with banana, milk, a handful of oats and a blender. It's as good as porridge and it will fill you up really well to get you through the morning.

Eat little and often

But not lots and often. I don't know about you, but I was brought up on three square meals a day, and told 'you shouldn't eat between meals'. Well, it turns out this isn't so (yippee!). You actually need to eat every three or four hours to keep your blood sugar level stable. If this level drops too far, you'll get an urge to eat – preferably something sweet – in order to give you energy. And that's when you head for the biscuit tin...

There's some research to show that people who eat several times throughout the day are slimmer than those who eat just a couple of meals. And more research, incidentally, suggesting that snacking throughout the day can help lower cholesterol. In other words, a mid-morning and mid-afternoon snack will actually help you lose weight.

But not if you're snacking on doughnuts. Or cheese sandwiches, Danish pastries, biscuits, chip butties, ice cream, or even a Stilton and walnut salad, or a bowl of soup. Make sure your snacks are low in calories and of modest proportions. A piece of fresh fruit is more like it, or a handful of dried fruit, or a low fat yoghurt. Keep it light and you'll find you're much less tempted to eat things you shouldn't between meals.

Watch those portions

Remember how those calories add up over a year? If you eat 100 calories a day more than you need to – that's a banana, say, or five squares of chocolate – you'll gain 10 lb a year (or have to burn that off extra). This means that it's really important to keep your portion sizes down to the right level.

It's so easy to put a little bit extra on your plate, or have a large handful of nuts instead of a small one, but it will make all the difference. Make sure you know how much of all your regular foods to eat. Even healthy foods contain calories, as you know.

The next few pages include a few strategies to help you follow this general principle, so there's no excuse for overeating by mistake. Calories you ingest by mistake still count, more's the pity.

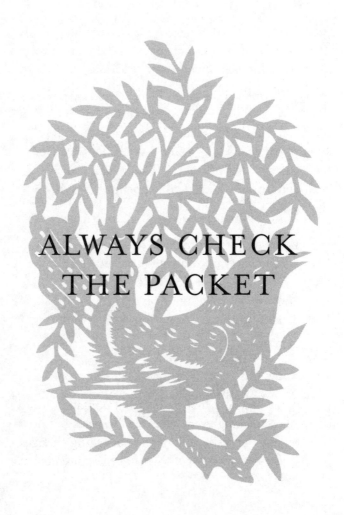

ALWAYS CHECK
THE PACKET

It's scary how portion sizes are increasing over the years. You may not realise it but there are now more calories in many standard foods than there used to be. Did you know that a medium slice of white bread now weighs 33 per cent more than it did 20 years ago? Ready-meals can now be as much as double the size they were back then too. Standard sizes of biscuits or cake slices are often bigger now, and so are portions of fast food and helpings in cafés and restaurants. Plenty of everyday products contain more calories than they used to, from Rice Krispies to Dairylea Triangles.

As manufacturers reformulate food, so their calorie content changes. Maybe they've upped certain ingredients in order to keep the flavour despite reducing the salt content. Maybe they've just increased the size of the tin or packet.

So don't assume anything. If it matters, check the packet and see how many calories it contains. You'd go mad rechecking every week just in case, but do keep an eye out, especially if the packaging changes in any way – it might be a clue that the contents have changed too.

Divide

your

cheese

When you buy something such as a lump of cheese, cut it up into 25 g/1 oz pieces as soon as you unpack the shopping. That way you know how much you're eating each time without having to guess, which is of course a thoroughly unreliable approach. If you use a calorie-counting method of losing weight (which makes sense), you can establish how many calories there are in each portion and then you know exactly what you're eating.

This can work for other things as well as cheese, of course. The point is that once you've made the effort once, the job's done. Otherwise, sooner or later, you'll be too lazy to measure it out properly. Besides, it's much easier to cut a 200 g lump into eight equal portions before you've started eating it.

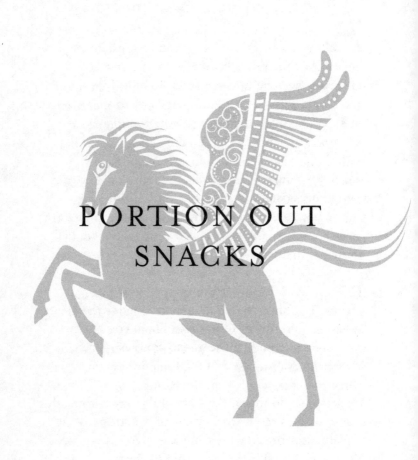

PORTION OUT
SNACKS

As well as dividing up cheese, and other regular cooking ingredients, you can also sort your snacks into portions. It can be sensible to make sure you always have 100-calorie snacks, whatever the weight of the food. I know, I know, I said I wasn't going to talk calories. But this way, once you've sorted out the portions you don't have to think about them again.

If you buy yourself nuts, or crisps,[1] or strawberries,[2] or yoghurt-coated raisins, weigh them into 100-calorie portions and put them into separate pots or bags. That way you can just grab one when you feel peckish, safe in the knowledge that you know what you're eating.

It's easy to kid yourself that healthy foods aren't fattening, and this process should help you avoid the trap of pretending there's no calories in fruit or vegetables.

You can also do this at the start of the day with fresh snacks such as raw carrot or cucumber sticks. Do it straight after breakfast if you have time – if you're feeling full you'll be less tempted to cheat.

[1] What do you think you're doing? You're supposed to be on a diet...
[2] That's better!

RECOGNISE
100 CALORIES

If you're going to think in portions of 100 calories for snacks, which is useful, it will help to have an idea of what constitutes 100 calories. Here are a few examples of snacks that come in at around that level:

- A piece of fruit
- Ten crisps
- Two oatcakes
- Half a snack-size Snickers bar
- One mini muffin
- Twenty almonds, peanuts or cashews
- Eight dried apricots
- Half a small avocado
- Two rice cakes with cottage cheese.

You can see from this not only how easy it would be to eat more than you realise if you don't measure it out, but also how much more satisfied some snacks will make you feel than others. Half an avocado or ten crisps? I'll take the avocado, thanks.

FIND A SHORTCUT

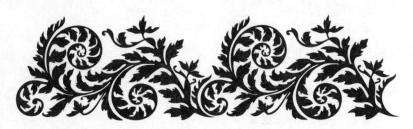

Laziness is often your chief enemy when it comes to portions. You can't be bothered to weigh out the rice because you can tell by looking when you've used the right amount. But actually, you only have to overestimate slightly every time you cook rice, for example, and you'll notice the difference when you stand on the scales.

One group of researchers found that if they asked people to take enough pasta out of a packet to feed two people, they took more if the packet was bigger. Which just goes to show that judging it by eye isn't reliable.

The way round this one is to weigh the right amount first time, and then to find a suitable container that will hold it. A plastic tub of some kind, or a cup, or a yoghurt pot, or whatever. Now mark with a permanent marker the level that your exact portion comes to. Every time you cook rice, you can measure it accurately without having to weigh it. Clever, huh? And no more excuses for cooking too much.

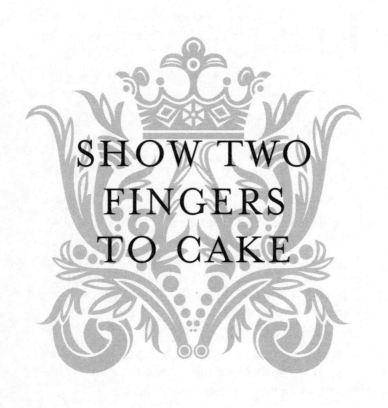

SHOW TWO
FINGERS
TO CAKE

No, you'll be pleased to hear I'm not suggesting you should never eat cake. I mean, that might be ideal but this is the real world. Sooner or later you'll want to try a bit of your child's birthday cake, or a sliver of gateau when you're having dinner with a friend. And the aim here is not to be miserable, so I'm not going to tell you never to eat cake.[1]

However (yes, there has to be a 'but'), we're going to have to do this in moderation. So I'm going to tell you how much cake you should allow yourself if you want to have your cake and eat it, so to speak. Think in terms of a slice of cake the width of two fingers – that's *at the widest end*, before you ask. Obviously I'm assuming the cake is average size and being cut into wedges. If not, use this as a guide and adapt it as necessary.

[1] And I'm not *that* big a hypocrite.

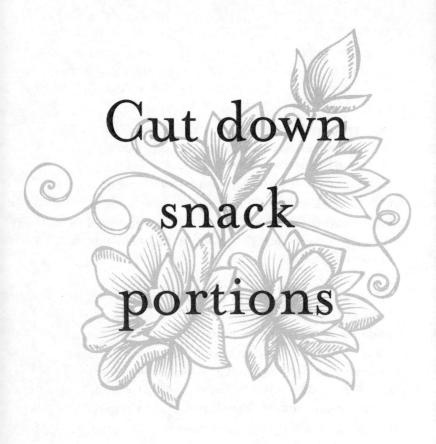

Cut down snack portions

One of the hardest things to give up can be your regular snack. If you always have a couple of biscuits with your mid-morning coffee, or a bar of chocolate when you fill up the car, the psychological effort required to give this up can seem insurmountable. You could of course give up the coffee, or abandon the car and take the train. But it's far better to find a way to wean yourself off the snack relatively painlessly.

And that's the trick – if you can't go cold turkey,[1] don't worry. Just take it in stages. Cut down to one biscuit instead of two, or go for a lower calorie chocolate bar (there are loads of websites that give the calorie content for chocolate bars rather than you having to pick all of them up and read the small print on the packet). If you find one biscuit feels wrong, break it in half so you still have two, they're just smaller. Or buy a brand with fewer calories.

Once you feel OK with this reduced snack – and you've proved to yourself that you can do this – you can now reduce it again. Or swap it to something healthier. Maybe you could have a banana with your coffee, or one of those low calorie health bars at the petrol station instead of the chocolate.

Depending on what else you're eating and what weight loss you're aiming for, this may be sufficient. If not, you can eventually wean yourself off the lower calorie snack too. You could even swap to something you don't much like so it's less of a wrench to give it up.

[1] Which you are allowed…

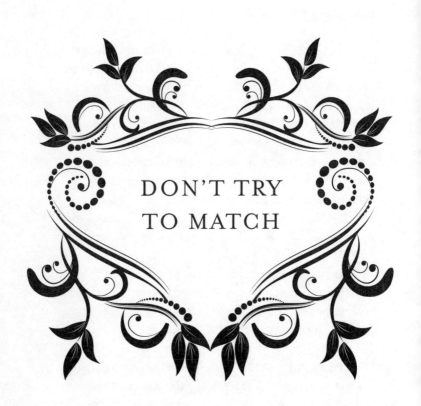

DON'T TRY
TO MATCH

Here's one that tends to be worse for women than for men. If you have a male partner, it's easy to cook a meal and then share it out equally between the two of you. But you should be consuming around 500 fewer calories than your partner, so you'll end up putting on as much as 1 lb a week like this.

Some men struggle with this too, of course. Whether you're dishing up the same portion for yourself as for your rugby-playing teenage son, or whether you're trying to match your mates pint for pint down the pub.

Do you know, recent research at Harvard University suggests that if a woman's best friend puts on weight, she is 57 per cent more likely to do the same thing? That's because we look to our friends to set acceptable behaviour, so if your friend has a slice of cake, you have one too.

What's the answer? Well, being aware of it is a big part. Dishing up more for some members of the family than for others will help too. And try not to meet for meals with friends who overeat – go to the cinema instead.

Eat less,
do more

I said you could lose weight without being miserable. We all know that the more we exercise the faster we'll lose weight, and please don't let me stop you if you want to join the gym or take up power walking. That's brilliant, and many ex-sluggards have found they love exercise when they find the right thing for them.

However, there are some of us who just don't enjoy it. Or who might enjoy it but don't have the time. Most people who say they haven't the time could make time if they really wanted to, but some people really can't. So you need to find ways to increase your calorie output even if you're not going to take up additional exercise. There are some suggestions over the next few pages, but you know your own life best and if you put your mind to it you can come up with some ideas of your own.

Ninety per cent of successful dieters exercise for about an hour a day. Mind you, they might not be doing step aerobics or training for a marathon. They may just be giving the dog a good long walk.

Know how much you're burning

R ight. I know all that calorie counting is tedious, and I know I said we'd stop doing it, but I lied. The fact is, you don't have to do it every time you eat or use up calories, but you do need a general overview of what calories are going in and out. And one of the things you need an idea of is how many calories you're burning.

Suppose you think to yourself, 'I can afford to eat this chocolate bar; after all I've just spent half an hour walking the dog.' Are you right? Setting aside the fact that if you pass on the chocolate bar you'll lose more weight than if you eat it, regardless of the dog walking, does a half hour walk actually equate to a chocolate bar's worth of calories?

So just to help you along, here's a list of how many calories you burn in half an hour of various activities. Obviously this isn't exact – I don't know how fast you walk your dog, and whether you stopped, and how vigorously you threw sticks for it. But it's a useful general guide.

Sleeping	35	Gardening	210
Sitting still	40	Dancing	230
Standing	45	Swimming	235
Driving	80	Tennis	235
Shopping	90	Football	270
Brushing your teeth	95	Walking up stairs	310
Cooking	100	Cycling	335
Yoga	110	Martial arts	390
Housework	110	High impact	400
Weight lifting	130	aerobics	
Walking	170	Running	700

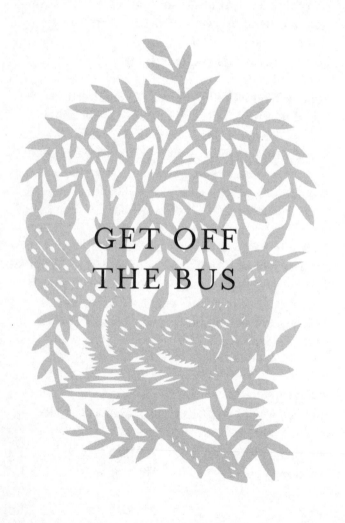

GET OFF
THE BUS

Walking is one of the best and easiest forms of exercise, which you can incorporate into your daily life without having to go somewhere different, find an extra hour, or squeeze into some daft lycra outfit.

All you have to do is get off the bus or train a stop earlier and walk the extra distance. Or park further away and walk. Whether it's work or the shops or school or visiting your mum, if you ever go anywhere you can do this.

As time goes on you can start getting off two stops early, or parking even further away. This is a level of exercise anyone should be able to find time for, and it really will help. At a reasonably brisk speed you can burn up 100 calories in 20 minutes (it depends on your weight and height – that's just approximate). And it's good for you in all sorts of other ways too.

Walk

faster

The faster you walk, the more calories you burn up. Suppose, given your weight and height, you walk for ten minutes at 2 mph (that's a gentle stroll) and burn up 26 calories. Well, if you double your speed to a brisk 4 mph you'd burn up 61 calories. That's more than double.

So even if you don't do any additional exercise at all, if you simply walk faster every time you walk – round the shops, out with the dog, to the office – you'll burn off more calories. The example above supposed you were only walking for ten minutes. What if it was half an hour? You'd burn an extra 100 calories just by speeding up.

Just one thing here – these figures are for equivalent times spent walking. If by walking at twice the speed you simply arrive in half the time, you've not gained. This is something to practise when the amount of walking isn't finite – for example, walking the dog or going round the park with the kids.

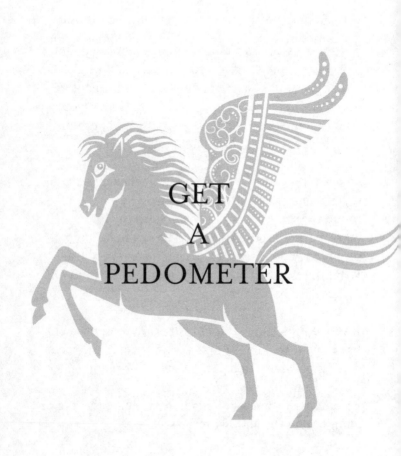

GET
A
PEDOMETER

If you're remotely serious about burning off more calories by walking, get yourself a pedometer. You know, one of those things that counts your steps and tells you how far you've walked. Some of them give you loads of information, but it's the step-counter bit that's the most useful.

If you want to be fit and healthy, you should aim to walk around 10,000 steps a day. That's equivalent to about five miles. I know that sounds scary, but remember you may be covering quite a lot of ground up and down the stairs at work, or pottering round the house doing the laundry. You won't reach that target figure without some dedicated walking of course, but you don't have to go on a five-mile hike every day.

If the idea of walking 10,000 steps seems unattainable to you, just start by finding out how many steps you walk at the moment. Then aim to increase it by, for example, 500 steps a day. Once you're used to that level of activity, add another 500 a day. Before you know it you'll be walking 10,000 steps a day, which will burn off roughly 500 calories.

MAKE
EVERYDAY LIFE
MORE
ENERGETIC

Quite apart from finding ways to add exercise to your life, you can also make your existing exercise more energetic. For example, since I started to lose weight I've made it a rule that I always run up stairs. Once that became easy, I took to running up them two at a time.

I have a friend who likes to cook to dance music. She dances as she makes her way around the kitchen and burns off extra energy that way. I also know someone who has a policy of always walking around the kitchen when she's on the phone. If you go to work on the train you may have to use an escalator. So make it a rule that you'll always walk up it and not stand still while it does all the work.

It doesn't matter how pushed for time you are, you can always find time for this kind of additional exercise. And every little helps.

MIND HOW
YOU PARTY

Social events do make it harder to lose weight. If you only get to go out once every few weeks it's not such a big deal, but if you socialise a lot, or go to loads of business functions, or start partying in early December and put on weight before you even get to Christmas, you need a few strategies to get you through.

You can let yourself go a bit if this really is a one-off, but the danger lies in thinking it's OK to let yourself go as a treat when, in fact, you have two or three similar treats a week. So the crucial thing is to be realistic about the scale of the risk, and if there's enough socialising to put weight on you, don't keep letting yourself off the hook.

Consciously make a point of working out how you're going to get through each party or event before you go to it. Think through what the likely temptations will be, and how you're going to address them without ruining your evening. The next few pages have some ideas, and always be on the lookout for others, or ask friends who are watching their weight how they cope with the social whirl. It can be done – trust me – it just takes a bit of thought.

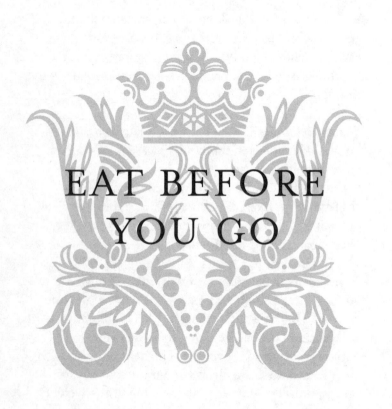

EAT BEFORE
YOU GO

I know this sounds daft. How is eating twice instead of once going to help? Well, the idea is that if you have a light snack before you go out, you'll be less hungry and it will be easier to moderate your eating once you arrive at the party. The 'light snack' is important here – this isn't going to work if you have a three-course meal before you go out.

If you're going to be having a sit-down meal, you don't want to be starving by the time it arrives (which may be later than your usual eating time). You'll just scoff down far more than you need before you notice whether you've had enough. If it's a buffet arrangement, it's far easier to resist the canapés if you've already had something to eat.

So whatever the occasion, eating a little something before you go, to take the edge off your hunger, will help you eat less once you get there.

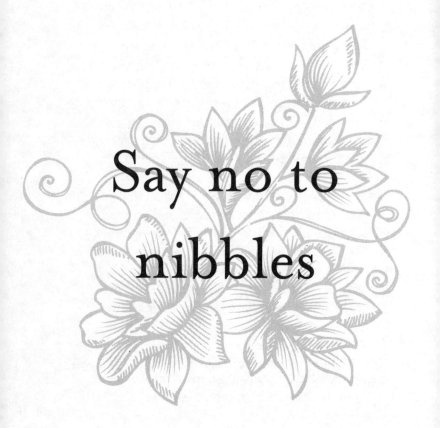

Say no to
nibbles

Those scrummy canapés and bowls of nuts are dangerous. You feel you're hardly eating, but you can put away a whole day's worth of calories in minutes. Just don't do it.

It's far easier not to start on the nibbles than to have a couple and then stop. If you really trust yourself, have two of the lightest looking canapés, with little or no pastry, and then stop. Or one modest handful of nuts or crisps. Then again, if you really trust yourself, why are you having any at all? Ideally, don't eat any of them – the trick here is not to look at them. If someone is bringing them round, make eye contact with the waiter as you say 'Not for me thanks' and have a competition with yourself to see if you can get through the evening without ever knowing what the canapés were. That will include not watching longingly as the person you're talking to lifts their food to their mouth.

Here's another quick tip. Don't stand anywhere near the buffet table or a bowl of nuts or anything else of the kind. It's so easy to eat mindlessly as you chat. Whereas if you're on the other side of the room it's almost impossible to graze.

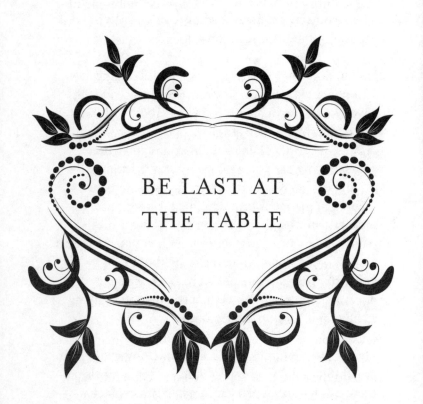

BE LAST AT
THE TABLE

If you're watching your weight at a buffet, you can gain advantage from the fact that you'll be one of the only people who is. Make sure you're one of the last to go up to the table, and chances are a lot of the high calorie food will have gone.

Bear in mind that although you might think salad isn't fattening, it's not true that all cold food is low in calories (it's an easy mistake to make, I know). There's nothing low calorie about pasta salad held together with mayonnaise, or cheese and bacon quiche. You want to go for salads that are high in fruit and vegetables and low on dressings. Cold chicken beats game pie, and you should choose the leanest slice of ham.

And watch the size of the plates too. If they're large, don't pile the plate high as well. Make sure you eat the same amount as you would if you were cooking sensibly for yourself at home. You might feel you're missing out as you reluctantly pass on that delicious creamy cheese flan, or the warm bread rolls, but go over to the other side of the room to eat it and enjoy what you have on your plate. You'll soon forget what you're going without, apart from being left with a well-deserved, warm virtuous feeling at the end of the evening.

Have two
starters

No, not as well as your main course... If you're eating out at a restaurant, one of the easiest ways to keep the calories down is to have a second starter when everyone else is eating their main course. Yes, it does have to be normal size and not main course-sized I'm afraid.

Personally I often find the starter list more appealing than the main courses, and frequently can't choose between a couple of them. So getting to eat two of them is quite a treat. If you think you might hate to forego some of those options for a main course, just don't read that part of the menu. By the time your friends' food has arrived it will be too late to change your mind.

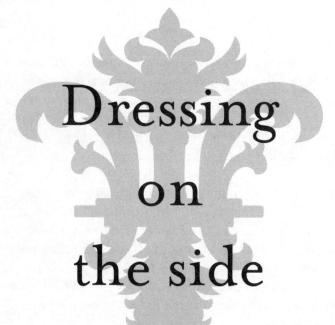

Dressing on the side

If you're ordering a salad, beware of all the calories in the dressing. I'm not suggesting you eat it without dressing altogether (unless you want to), but you'll save a lot of calories if you can avoid most of the dressing.

The way round this is to ask the waiter to serve the dressing on the side. One option is to allow yourself just one or two dessertspoons of dressing and drizzle them over the salad yourself. Or you can leave the dressing where it is and dip your salad into it as you eat.

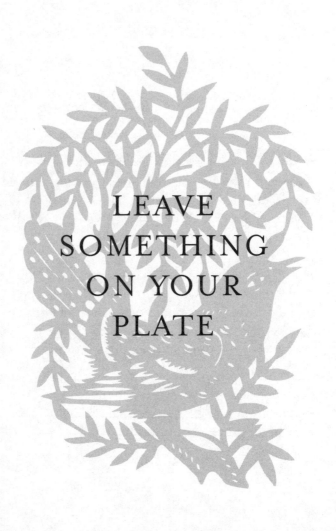

LEAVE
SOMETHING
ON YOUR
PLATE

Believe it or not, if you leave a quarter of your food on your plate, you can save 300 calories on an average restaurant meal. Obviously I haven't gone round and done all the research myself, but this was a statistic that really struck me when I read it.

I should point out that this isn't going to be hugely helpful if you leave all the lettuce and eat the rest. Try leaving the potatoes, or part of the main dish, or the pastry off the top of the pie.[1] That will really make a worthwhile difference.

Generally speaking it's a good idea to order food that comes without sauce as that's where the calories often hide. So grilled fish is far lower in calories than fish in any kind of sauce. If you do succumb to the temptations of a dish with a rich sauce, aim to leave plenty of the sauce on your plate.

---

[1] I know it's the best bit. All right, just leave half the pastry then.

Share the pudding round

O f course the very best, most abstemious option is to go without pudding, and most of the time it's best if you can manage to do this. However, if you're not trying to drop three clothing sizes but just want to break even weight-wise, it seems a shame to skip pudding every time you go out.

If you're out with other friends or a partner who feels the same, why not order one pudding for the whole table to share? After all, by this stage in the proceedings no one is actually hungry. It's just that you want to taste the pudding because it sounds so good.

So, if you decide not to skip straight on to coffee this time, the only challenge is agreeing with your companions which pudding to order between you.

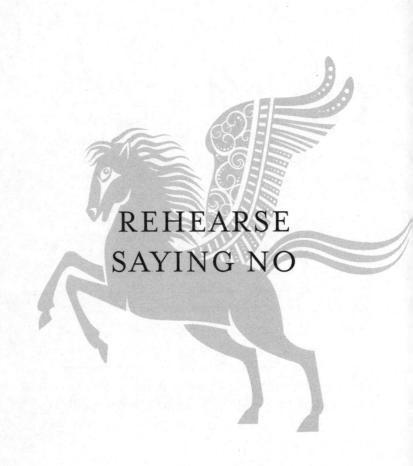

REHEARSE
SAYING NO

I know someone who lost four stone in a year. He didn't go on any specific diet, he just cut out bread, potatoes, puddings and so on. He was in fact rather fond of his puddings, and when he went out for business lunches – as he quite often did – he had trouble resisting.

His ingenious solution to this was to practise in advance, ready for when the waiter came round to take the pudding order, saying, 'Just coffee for me thanks.' This became so natural that he found it came out of his mouth before he'd had a chance to think about it.

If you know what your danger points are – and I bet you do – just rehearse the 'correct' answer, in front of a mirror if you like, so that when the time comes you can make the response you know you want to.

COOK YOUR OWN

I know it's not always possible to prepare your own food, especially when you're socialising, but only if you cook it yourself do you really know what's in it. Anyone else might have put in twice the mayonnaise you would have done, or used full fat Greek yoghurt, or fried it instead of grilling.

If you want to control your food intake, do your best to control the cooking. Invite friends to eat with you instead of the other way round (especially if they tend to cook rich food). Make your own packed lunch for work instead of buying something at the local sandwich bar. Meet friends for coffee instead of lunch (unless you're cooking it).

I used to tell myself I had too busy a lifestyle to cook for myself very often, but when I really put my mind to losing weight I found it was possible to prepare my own food much more often than I'd previously pretended to myself. In the end it comes down to how much you really want to shift the weight. If you care enough, you'll find a way.

LIMIT THE
ALCOHOL

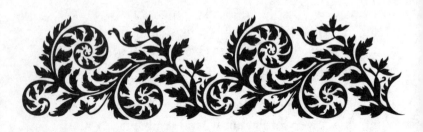

Clearly one of the most high calorie components of any social event for lots of people is the alcohol. You may have successfully cut down your drinking at home, but it's much harder when you're surrounded by friends who are drinking whatever they like.

There are certainly some drinks that are lower calorie than others. Wines and spirits have fewer calories per serving than beers and lagers, so they're your best bet (so long as you don't drink twice as many servings). Best of all are white wine spritzers – or indeed any kind of watered down wine – where the amount of wine in the glass is reduced.

Another option is to alternate water and alcohol through the evening. If you make every other drink water, this will also be healthy, fill you up more, help keep you sober, and – if you go beyond that point – still hugely reduce the risk of a hangover next morning. So why wouldn't you?

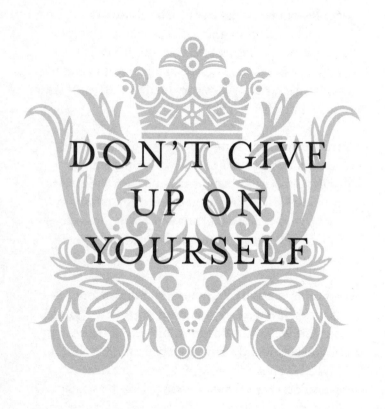

DON'T GIVE
UP ON
YOURSELF

I tried to give up smoking several times. Once I even managed it for eight months, but in the end I went back to the fags. Eventually, however, after decades of smoking, I did give up successfully.[1] The thing about giving up smoking is that just because you can't do it this time, that doesn't mean you won't be able to do it next time. You just need to find the way that works for you.

And the same goes for losing weight. I battled unsuccessfully with my weight for years before I found the motivation to lose it. Then the combination of the right time and the right strategies did the trick. Just because the last diet didn't work, or the one before that, it doesn't mean the next one won't.

The important thing is not to get too hung up on the diet itself but to do the work inside your head. And if you have a bad day or a bad week – or even a bad couple of years – it doesn't mean you'll never lose the weight. You just haven't lost it yet.

So don't give up. Think positive. Use the strategies in this book, and work on what's going on inside your head rather than your stomach, and it's only a matter of time before you'll be as slim as you want to be.

[1] So far, anyway. And it's been several years now.

More titles by Richard Templar …

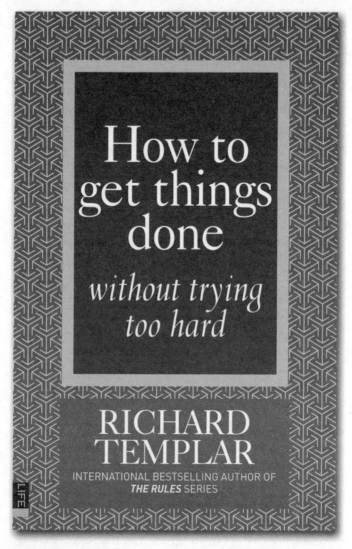

ISBN 9780273725565

A preview of How to get things done without trying too hard …

Turn your toothbrush upside down

When I was young I was always told that if I wanted to remember something I should put a knot in my handkerchief. Well, trouble is that no one really carries a handkerchief any more (except maybe great aunts). I've tried knotting a tissue but they just tear. However, there are other ways to remember things.

If I think of something at bedtime that I mustn't forget in the morning, I turn my toothbrush upside down. This might sound daft, but I know I'll use my toothbrush in the morning, and I'll look at it and think, "What on earth is that doing upside down?" Then I'll remember. And yes, I always do remember[1]. The trick is that as you turn it over you have to visualise yourself doing whatever it is – taking the cat to the vet, or putting the CD in your briefcase, or taking the meringues out of the oven. That way, you'll know in the morning what you were supposed to remember.

Of course there are other ways of using this trick. You can hang your bag or jacket on a different hook to remind you when you leave that your mobile isn't in it because it's on charge. Or put an upside down pudding basin in the middle of the kitchen table to signify that the plants need watering. In fact, you can be as quirky as you like, because the important thing is that when you next look at the thing, you need to think, "What on earth…?"

[1] Of course I may have forgotten again before I actually get to do whatever it is, but that's another matter.

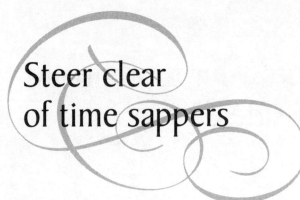

Steer clear
of time sappers

Some things just eat up time. The most obvious one, as I've mentioned, is the Internet. I don't want to knock it because I know it's a brilliant invention, makes all our lives easier etc etc, but it can waste as much time as it saves if you let it.

We all have our own time sappers. Backgammon is one of mine. Once I start playing I don't know where the time goes. Electronic toys from Playstations to Wii are common ones, and others don't involve playing at all. Some people spend hours in the kitchen, cooking things that taste delicious but take ages, when they're quite capable of whipping up something just as delicious in a fraction of the time. I know people who spend hours cleaning when frankly a quick vacuum round would have done the job. And then there are time sappers in people form – the ones who you simply can't have a quick chat with because it always turns into two hours or more, when you least have two hours to spare.

When you're not pressed for time, of course all these things are fine. But if you want to get more done you'll need to learn where your time goes and be firm about the time sappers. By far the best approach is to steer clear altogether. Save them for when your time isn't limited, and while you're busy give them a wide berth.

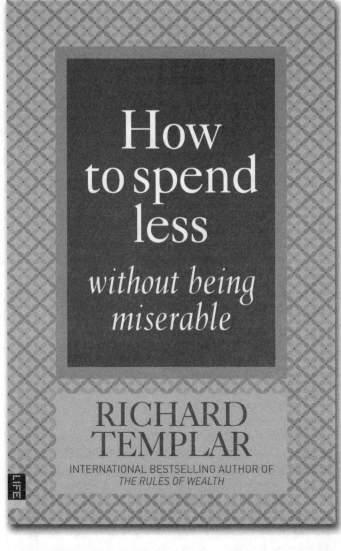

How
to spend
less

*without being
miserable*

RICHARD
TEMPLAR

INTERNATIONAL BESTSELLING AUTHOR OF
THE RULES OF WEALTH

ISBN 9780273725558

Turn the page for a preview …

Buy at auction

I know, it's that scary worry that you'll develop a nervous tic and find you've bought a priceless artwork for millions[1], when all you wanted was a box of assorted second-hand crockery for a fiver. But it's worth getting over the nerves because you can save a lot of money at auction, especially for bigger items such as cars, computers, electrical goods, houses and land.

The crucial thing is to set your maximum price in advance and then not to go above it. You need to be absolutely clear about how much the thing is worth to you, and set your level accordingly. And of course to have done your research thoroughly - both checking out the item and the market value. Of course you know that you must be very disciplined, clearly identify what you want first, and if you don't get it at your pre-decided price be ready to walk – not buy something else to fill the disappointment void.

If you really don't trust yourself not to get carried away, the foolproof way round this is to get someone else to go along and bid on your behalf, having told them what price they're not to exceed. I say foolproof – obviously if you ask an excitable and impulsive optimist to do this for you you may get what you deserve. But ask someone careful and level-headed and you'll be entirely safe.

[1] I've never understood how something priceless can have a price

Stick to tap water

Do you have any idea how much you spend on bottled water? Work it out – go on. Alright I'll give you a clue. If you drink one litre a day, it's costing you around £260 a year, depending on the brand obviously. And if you drink more than that, you can do the calculations yourself. Likewise if you buy it in cafés or restaurants it will be costing you far more. In fact, bottled water in the UK costs about as much as petrol[1].

And that's before you start considering the impact on the environment of bottled water in almost every way – production, packaging and transport.

Now think what you could be doing with that money instead. You could feed your family for an extra fortnight or more, go out for the evening several times, do a good chunk of your Christmas shopping, buy your mum flowers every month… oh, all sorts of things. Even if they're just boring but important things like being able to pay the bills. You could even buy yourself a water filter if you really don't like the idea of drinking water straight from the tap, and a reusable bottle to take it with you everywhere.

And if you're thinking, "Ah, but I can't get fizzy water out of the tap, can I?" you'd be right. But you can buy a water carbonator and still have change from all the money you'll save.

[1] And you would't drink that, would you?

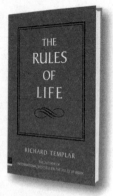
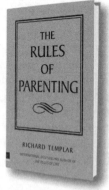
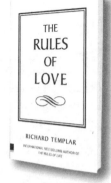
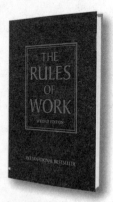
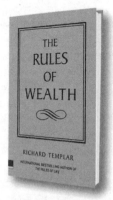
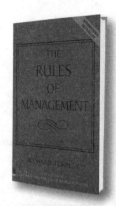